Curing Electromagnetic Hypersensitivity

© Copyright: Steven Magee 2014

Edition 2 - Published 2015

Cover Picture: From top to bottom we can see the "Ring of Fire" solar eclipse in process, an internal camera reflection of the solar eclipse and a hang glider that was flying in the area. Electromagnetic Hypersensitivity (EHS) sufferers are commonly affected by changes in natural electromagnetic radiation levels from solar eclipses, solar flares and sunspots.

Contents

Introduction

Curing Electromagnetic Hypersensitivity was a book that took five years to develop. I became aware that I was displaying the symptoms of Radio Wave Sickness in 2009 after commissioning a very large utility solar photovoltaic power plant. What I was not aware of at that time was extended time in the Radio Wave Sickness state can lead to the development of Electromagnetic Hypersensitivity in the human.

Everyone will show some of the symptoms of Radio Wave Sickness when in high powered radio wave fields. This was proven back in the 1930's. Raise the radio wave levels sufficiently high enough and you will start to kill people. It is the reason why the Federal Communications Commission (FCC) exists. They have set limits on radio frequency power levels in an effort to prevent this. However, as we know today, their limits are far too high. This has allowed the overloading of the human environment with radio waves that are now known to be biologically harmful to a subset of the general population.

The longer a person is in a man-made radio wave field, the more likely it is that they will progress into the Electromagnetic Hypersensitivity state. What happens when you cross over from Radio Wave Sickness and into Electromagnetic Hypersensitivity? It will feel like you have transitioned into outer Space and are not wearing the protective spacesuit. Previously tolerated radio wave exposures will become intolerable. Your home and office environments will become hostile to you. Cities and towns will make you sick and the only respite from that sickness is found in the remote countryside. People who progress into extreme Electromagnetic Hypersensitivity become nomadic, unable to tolerate any location for long periods of time. Unfortunately, some of these people eventually commit suicide due to their deteriorating health.

The deployment of cell phone towers over the last few decades, the adoption of cell phones by the masses, Wi-Fi, wireless devices and the installation of radio frequency transmitting utility meters has brought this sickness into the lives of many people. It is sold to the modern masses as "Progress"; to the electro-sensitives, it is biological warfare. Why are corporations waging environmental terrorism on these people? Because they can. Corporate and government electronic harassment is an "Inconvenient Truth" that currently very few places in the world are addressing.

Having experienced the degradation of health from Radio Wave Sickness into the Electromagnetic Hypersensitivity state and managed to clear up the extreme sensitivity, there was a need to publish the research and techniques that I used. This book details my experiences and how I developed the methods that I used to continue living in modern society.

The techniques are not unique to Radio Wave Sickness and Electromagnetic Hypersensitivity, but also may be applied to a myriad of other health conditions. Conditions that are suspected to have links to electromagnetic exposures are:

- Poor circulation.

- Skin changes.

- Tremors.

- Headaches and migraines.

- Seizures.

- Heart disorders.

- Diabetes.

- Fatigue.

- Asthma.

- Allergies.

- Food sensitivities or intolerance.

- Memory fog.

- Autism.

- Attention Deficit Disorder (ADD).

- Hyperactivity.
- Alzheimer's.
- Parkinson's.
- Dementia.
- Multiple Sclerosis (MS).
- Lou Gehrig's (ALS).
- Multiple Chemical Sensitivity (MCS).
- Cancer.
- Triggering of the human mating cycle.

If you are seeing any of the above or have strange health conditions that your doctor cannot diagnose, then you may find this book enlightening. Electromagnetic radiation exposures are diverse and can create an equally diverse range of reactions in the human.

This book is aimed at the general public, the medical profession and the engineering profession. Mathematics is avoided and the book presents the concepts of the various forms of health in a readable format to the general public. Important points are in bold font.

This book contains the very latest research on health and the human environment. It should be viewed as the current ideas and the contents are subject to review by the scientific community. The author and publisher accept no liability whatsoever for any of the contents and the book is published in the spirit of unrestricted access to the latest ideas and scientific theories in a changing world.

You should always consult with a licensed and certified medical professional on any aspects of health, sickness or disease.

"We are all modern day explorers of an invisible alien world."

Steven Magee CEng MIET BEng Hons

United Kingdom

I started to play around with electricity when I was thirteen years old. Around that time I got my first home computer system which was to spark an interest in electricity and electronics. I left school at sixteen and became an apprentice electrician at the city center university research and teaching hospital. I worked in the electrical group for ten years and I have to say that I noticed people changing during that time.

I had noticed that some of the electricians had made the electrical rooms into workshops and they spent most of their day in them. In particular, there were two electricians who used to take their breaks in these rooms and sleep against the switchgear. They had very strange personalities!

In 1987 the hospital was in the process of switching over from conventional florescent lighting to electronic florescent lighting and installing computer systems for the medical records. There were robots in the sterile areas, ultrasonic baths, high frequency induction furnaces in the laboratories, RADAR operated automatic doors, and so on. I was working with many modern devices and no one ever warned me about the toxicity of these. In fact, no one ever told me about effects such as stray voltage, electromagnetic radiation health effects, harmonic energy making electromagnetic fields on cables get very large, pulsating magnetic fields affecting the brain, electrical and electronic field emissions and to stay out of them.

I would regularly walk through the hospital underground distribution system corridors and be inches from 6,600 volt AC electricity power cables and florescent lights. We would smash up the numerous florescent tubes that we would change every week, releasing toxic clouds of mercury contaminated white phosphor dust. Today, I can only imagine what these things must have been doing to my biological health!

The thing about working in a hospital is that you get to meet a lot of people who are sick and dying. I would have

many conversations with these people over the years. The consistent thing that they would repeatedly say to me was they could not understand how they had become ill. It was always a mystery to them.

It is interesting that in 1987 Dr. John Nash Ott had actually published all of his research into electromagnetic radiation:

- My Ivory Cellar; [The Story of Time-Lapse Photography]. 1958.

- Health and Light: The Extraordinary Study That Shows How Light Affects Your Health and Emotional Well Being. 1973.

- Exploring the Spectrum: The Effects of Natural and Artificial Light on Living Organisms. 1975.

- Light, Radiation, and You: How to Stay Healthy. 1982.

- Color and Light: Their Effects on Plants, Animals and People. 1987.

Dr. John Nash Ott had discovered by 1987 that glass, artificial light sources, electricity and electronic systems were having extensive detrimental effects on plants, animals and humans. No one at the hospital was talking about it. The hospital had 1,000 beds, an animal research facility, a university research facility, a nursing teaching center, a doctors teaching center, a dental teaching center and on site residence buildings to house all of the students. It was a huge university campus! One can only wonder why no one was talking about the toxicity of light, electricity, electronic systems and wireless radiation.

As well as my day job, I would go to college and university one day and one night per week. I obtained an Ordinary National Certificate, Higher National Certificate, Higher National Diploma, and a Bachelors Degree with Honors in Electrical and Electronic Engineering. I can tell you that in ten years of studying electricity and electronics, not one mention was ever made of the toxicity of electricity.

Dr. John Nash Ott authored his last publication in 1987. I graduated in 1996, some nine years later. His work was never mentioned in any of my classes or text books on the subject. No teachings were given to me about the toxicity of electricity. Harmonics was taught, but only for its effects on electrical equipment, not human health. No mention was ever made about the very large electromagnetic fields that it puts onto cables and equipment.

One of the things that I remember as an apprentice was that when I started at the hospital, I was extremely fatigued for the first few months of working there. The mechanical apprentice who started at the same time as me was reporting the same thing. Today, I know that effect to be the body adjusting to toxic environmental conditions.

Both the mechanical apprentice and myself were from rural areas outside of the city. Working at a highly industrialized facility in the city center was an alien environment for us. In addition to the variety of modern equipment that the hospital had, it had a large number of telecommunications radio frequency transmission antenna systems on the roof. Today it is known that these systems are harmful to the human at close proximity. We were constantly working near the antenna systems with no precautions.

I had found the people in the facilities team to be mostly pleasant, but a little strange too. I had also noticed personalities changing during the ten years that I worked in this group, my own personality was also changing. In particular, I do remember one of the members of the electrical team being exceptionally friendly and very smart and he actually became the opposite, unfriendly and mean during the time I knew him. The adoption of electronics and computer systems into the hospital had become rampant during that time period. This particular person had a number of metal implants that today we know to be incompatible with exposure to the various forms of electricity.

I had noticed that my face was constantly flushing and that my memory was having issues. Forgetfulness was quite normal during my time there and I was always tired. My mating cycle was frequently being triggered and I thought it was normal. I had never known any different.

In 1996 I changed my position and started working with dialysis machines. These were highly complex computer controlled machines that were filled with the latest electrical and electronic products. The joke in the group was that everyone who joined the team got divorced shortly afterwords! Little did they know that it was the electromagnetic radiation emissions from the machines that was probably causing it.

I had noticed my health significantly degrading in my late twenties after joining this group. General aches and pains, feeling lethargic, nosebleeds, gums bleeding after brushing my teeth and being extremely tired in the mornings had become normal. Getting up in the mornings was always difficult. Working on my home during the weekends was a problem due to the low energy levels. I later realized that part of this may have been coming from drinking reverse osmosis water. The dialysis team was making its tea and coffee with the same reverse osmosis water that the machines used! Reverse osmosis water is highly processed water that is extremely mineral deficient!

It was the first position that had issued me with a laptop computer system, anti-static strap and pager. I remember seeing the doctor about recurring chapped lips that had shown up in this position and they told me it was normal. I now know that it was exposure to the artificial light from the laptop computer that was causing this. The pager was constantly clipped to my belt and would work throughout the region, so I know that I was in extensive unnatural radio fields that communicated with it. I would have the pager with me, even when I slept. I do wonder if the early pager systems had harmful biological emissions from them? I was also being exposed to stray voltage and stray frequencies from the anti-static strap which is extensively documented in the diary industry for making farmers, their families, and their animals sick.

The first person that I knew who committed suicide was in this group. I will always be curious to know if it was caused in part from the toxic exposures that he received during his time in it. He was in the group for many years, as opposed to the three years that I worked there.

"Never go to a doctor whose office plants have died."

Erma Bombeck

La Palma

In 1999 I went to live in La Palma in the Canary Islands and started to work at an altitude of approximately 7,755 feet. I was working with telescope drive systems that were controlled by industrial computer systems. There are no doubts that sunlight in the right dose is an excellent medication! Living in the Canary Islands did wonders for improving my health. However, it was short lived.

I noticed that the longer I was in the position in the Canary Islands, the sicker I was getting. Like many people in this situation, I did not understand what was happening. Today, I do believe that I was actually sitting in the fields of the neighbors cathode ray tube (CRT) television when I was at home. The problem with CRT televisions is that they have extensive fields around them and those fields will pass straight through walls! Their television was on the other side of the wall from my sofa.

I had also been issued with a laptop computer at work and I was constantly working on it. Email had become a popular form of communication. There were no warnings given about laptop computers and human health. I now know that many laptop computers have unnatural magnetic fields around them, emit electromagnetic interference, and that their displays can induce health problems into the human.

I purchased my first cellphone in La Palma. I had noticed after having it for a while that it would cause strange noises on my stereo system in the car. I now understand this to be the cellphone logging into the cellphone tower every ten minutes or so. The transmission was so powerful from the cellphone that it was interfering with the stereo system!

I lived in two properties in La Palma and the second property was a home that was in the countryside. I only lived in that home for a short period before leaving for my next position in Hawaii. However, I had noticed that my girlfriend was constantly complaining of headaches there and my health was continuing to decline. Today, I suspect that it was the street lights that were outside of the home. Many street lights create a toxic form of light to the human, create stray voltage/currents/frequencies, and they can have strange electromagnetic emissions from them.

"Epistemology has always been affected by technologies like the telescope and the microscope, things that have created a radical shift in how we sense physical reality."

Ken Goldberg

Hawaii

I moved to the USA in 2001 and lived in Waimea on the island of Hawaii. I was walking to and from work under the high voltage power lines that run through the streets there. During that time I had noticed that I was getting very anxious and that if I was placed in a stressful situation that my heartbeat would start to race and my face would flush. I attribute that health effect to the high voltage power lines, as it cleared up when I moved away from Waimea.

Working at approximately 13,796 feet is well known to be harmful to human health and most people on the mountain were in some state of sickness. We were commuting up and down the mountain daily and our bodies were constantly in a state of confusion. I knew from conversations with other staff members that poor health was a feature of daily high altitude commuting. Pilots, air hostesses, and frequent fliers suffer from the same thing.

At 13,796 feet very little grows! It is a barren landscape that is just rocks and cinder. When you work at high altitude you notice that trees stop growing at a very definite altitude. This line of demarcation is called the "Tree Line". It appears to be an effect of radiation exposure. As you increase in altitude, the air gets thinner and less solar radiation filtering is taking place. More energy is in the electromagnetic spectrum and it appears to move outside of what the trees can survive in. You will find very strange growth patterns in the trees near the tree line with unusual branching and weird deformities. For this reason, I advise people to be very careful with high altitude radiation exposure. If there are no trees around at altitude, then you should avoid the sunlight, as it may give you a very strange type of radiation sickness!

In Hawaii, I had a strange beach encounter with a group of people that I had started chatting to. It turned out that they were all having health problems and were in Hawaii to try and recover their health. They invited me into their oceanfront home

14

where there were a wide range of medical devices that they were using. Among the devices they had was a "Zapper" that applies pulsed DC voltage to the hands and an oxygen tent. Like many people, this group had watched their health mysteriously decline as they had aged. It was a mystery to them how they had ended up in poor health. Unfortunately, meeting them was like meeting myself a decade later, I just did not know it at the time.

In 2003, I joined the astronomy team and moved onto the night shift. I had suspected that living on the mountain for a week and having a week off would be healthier and it was! I also started to build a solar photovoltaic powered home in Hawaii. Everything was going well, until I moved into the home. The home was powered by a modified sine wave inverter that was running on high capacity 24 volt DC batteries that were charged by 8 solar photovoltaic modules. Like most off-grid homes, it had "Energy Star" compact florescent lighting (CFL) throughout the home.

I had noticed that there was a constant buzzing on the phone line whenever I would use it. I spoke with the electrician who had installed it and I was advised that it was a feature of off-grid homes. I was developing a wide variety of health issues the longer that I lived in the home. The main health symptom was fatigue. The longer I lived there, the more excessive the fatigue got. I got to the point where I would drink energy drinks and then go to bed and sleep. The drinks were having no effect on me! However, my mating cycle was constantly being triggered.

Today, I realize that the buzzing on the phone line was a combination of dirty electricity on the electrical grounding system combined with radio wave emissions from the electrical wiring. The effect was made worse during the night from the compact florescent lights (CFL) putting harmonics onto the electrical cables and the electromagnetic fields that they emit. I did not know it at the time, but I had developed Radio Wave Sickness (RWS)!

I knew two other people who lived in off-grid solar powered homes very well. One was extremely passive aggressive with most people and his personality was lacking empathy. The other was showing severe symptoms of forgetfulness. When you explore the field of dirty electricity, you find that the off-grid homes generally have the poorest power quality. The quality of electricity will vary with the loads on the system. It is likely that this dirty electricity was a source of their problems.

I developed intestinal pains during working on the night shift and about every two weeks I would get painful cramps that would lead to diarrhea. I did not know it at the time, but it is classical symptoms of shifting solar radiation exposure. It would generally occur on my first day off in sunlight after working a week of nights.

The visions were the most fascinating thing about working nights. It is very surreal to have to stop the car on your way down from the summit to your bedroom because a Hawaiian princess on a horse is in the road! You look all around and it is just the two of you and a horse in a barren lava field at 4 AM. You look away, you look back, they have gone and off to bed you go. The radioactivity from Space gets very high on top of these 13,796 feet mountain peaks and was likely a factor in these hallucinations. Unfortunately, working at approximately 13,796 feet is like working at a leaky nuclear reactor due to the radiation from Space!

The adverse health affects in people are well documented in the medical profession and by high altitude climbers. The advice is not to go to 13,796 feet in one day. Most of the observatories truck their staff from near sea level to the summit and back down every day! It makes many of them sick and they end up self medicating on the free company supplied drugs on the mountain. After several months they get the nasty drug side effects as well as the high altitude sickness. Many summit employees are walking around up there with medications in their pockets, such as aspirin and ibuprofen for the headaches, antacids for the stomach and sickness problems, and throat lozengers and cold medications for the sore throats and runny noses. The abnormal summit lifestyle eventually turns some of them into zombies and they end up arguing with each other. When I worked there, there was no disclosure of this to the new hires, other than *"You may get altitude sickness working here"*.

I saw two of the long term summit employees that I knew very well die during my time at the W. M. Keck Observatory from disease conditions. They each had spent approximately a decade working on the mountain. I was quite sick after working 5 years on the summit. Interestingly, my coworker at La Palma died from cancer after many years of high altitude work.

The second person that I knew who committed suicide had worked at the W. M. Keck Observatory for some years. He was a welder. Welders get exposed to significant levels of stray voltage, stray currents, stray frequencies, ultraviolet light and various electromagnetic radiation emissions from their arc welding equipment. Both of the people I have worked with who committed suicide were nice people. Unfortunately, it is well known that electromagnetic radiation exposures can make nice people do strange things that are out of character for them. The strange environmental radiation at these high altitude facilities does seem to have an impact on the staff, *"kooky"* as some people call it.

> *"The soul without imagination is what an observatory would be without a telescope."*
>
> *Henry Ward Beecher*

Arizona

In 2006 I changed jobs and went to live in Tucson, Arizona. This signified a move back onto normal utility electricity. The strange thing was, I had noticed the same effect occurring that I had noticed when I started working in the hospital. I was constantly fatigued in this position to the point of almost falling asleep every day in the first few months.

Kitt Peak is near to the Barry M. Goldwater Air Force Range where the military conduct bombing missions. This means that there are supersonic aircraft in the area and also the high powered sonic booms that they generate. The sonic booms are frequent, very noisy and make the buildings shake. I was quite surprised how powerful they were and no one had informed me of the known toxicity of sonic booms to the human. Wikipedia states: *"Some studies claim to show that sonic booms from U.S. Navy testing in Vieques, Puerto Rico, increased the incidence of vibroacoustic disease, a thickening of heart tissue."*

One of the notable things about Kitt Peak Observatory is the amount of lightning strikes that it gets during the monsoon season. There is a very high density of lightning strikes occurring on Kitt Peak mountain. It is the only place in the world that I have been to and actually seen lightning connect with a tree. It is an impressive sight to see the pulsations of white light from the forked lightning as it heats up the tree with a glowing red light. One of the most famous pictures of Kitt Peak shows the observatories on the peak surrounded by forked lightning. No one informed me that being in a high lightning environment is known to be hostile to human mental and physical health. Close exposure lightning has a wide range of electromagnetic radiation emissions from it.

I was living for the first six months that I was in Tucson in a place called Sabino Canyon. It has a very picturesque National Park. Every evening when I would come home from Kitt Peak, I would see lightning flashes inside the canyon. That year the canyon had its roads washed out by landslides and floods. It was an exceptional year for lightning storms. Unfortunately for me, it meant that not only was I being exposed to high intensity lightning at work, but it was also occurring at home! I was having crazy intestinal pains that were so bad that they would cause me to fall over at home. The doctor diagnosed me as having a twist in my intestines, however he never performed any diagnostics to come to this conclusion. It was as if he had made it up. What was really going on was the electromagnetic energy from the lightning storms was having profound effects on my intestinal system. The intense intestinal pains significantly subsided once monsoon season was over.

I was also spending four hours per day in transportation systems and eight hours at the observatory. We were driving next to high voltage power lines and passing close to high powered radio frequency transmitter systems. At the observatory I had measured the voltage waveform on the AC electrical system there and it was highly distorted. This distortion creates large amounts of harmonic energy on the AC electrical system and puts very large fields on the wiring and equipment. I did not realize the implications of that at the time, because I had never been taught that man-made electromagnetic radiation emissions and electrical system harmonics were harmful!

I remember when I saw it that I was surprised. Out at the telescope it was a highly distorted AC voltage sine wave. However, at the uninterruptible power supply (UPS), it was an almost perfect AC voltage sine wave. The sine wave got better the closer to the UPS system and worse the further away from it. I suspect that electronically generated AC voltage sine waves do not travel well over distances, particularly when they are feeding into electronic products. It is likely that the different frequencies of energy in electronically generated AC voltage sine waves start to interact with cables and the electronic products that they supply and this may distort them.

I later hired a contractor to assist with work at the observatory and it was not long before I was hearing the same story from him, he was getting really fatigued too! Today, I attribute the fatigue problems to the electromagnetic fields that were created by the harmonic energy on the AC electrical system.

At home, my relationship was problematic and within a year we had broken up. All I wanted to do was lay in bed, as my energy levels were so low. I could not sleep much, as I had insomnia constantly. I was getting intestinal pains and diarrhea a few times every month. I had to stop exercising in 2007 as I would get chest pains and breathing difficulties!

During my time in this position I had developed very strange facial and head pains. They would come and go and I had no idea what it was. I started to go to the doctor and was sent for many tests. No one could tell me what it was. During researching the book "Toxic Electricity", I realized that my seat at the office was next door to the telescope electrical room that contained all of the control systems, Wi-Fi router, networks, and computers! I was sitting next to a LASER printer and nearby was the cordless phone. I had been sitting in very large electromagnetic fields every day. The fact that my company wireless laptop computer also had large electromagnetic emissions coming out of it did not help.

The longer that I was in the position, the more aches and pains I was getting. My skin was getting to be so hot and painful that I was having daily baths to try and calm it down. The strange thing was, I looked perfectly normal on the outside! No one would have been aware that my health was failing. Insomnia was a big issue and it was rare that I would get a good nights sleep.

Anxiety became a significant problem and it was getting worse with time. My ability to manage the team was severely compromised and by the time that I left, I was having significant public speaking problems that were not present when I started the position. I knew I was being poisoned, I just could not figure out the source of the poison!

I later reported that I had identified a number of environmental health issues to the management team of this facility in 2012, after I had published the book "Toxic Electricity". I did not tell them what I had identified, as I was interested to see if they would want to know. Unfortunately, their response to the problems was silence. Responding with silence to inconvenient truths is a common problem in the workplace today and is a major problem with the prevalence of Sick Building Syndrome (SBS). Many managers know that their facilities are causing their staff to be sick, but stay silent about it. What I found most concerning about this is that it was an Ivy League college and university that specializes in human health!

I joined the solar industry in 2008 and by this time fatigue, insomnia, occasional intestinal pains and diarrhea, hot skin, and general aches and pains throughout my body had become something that I had accepted as aging. My doctor was informing me that it was a normal aspect of aging, everyone is the same! Staying awake on the job was getting to be a significant problem.

I eventually started to see the doctor for medication to keep me awake in order to keep working. I was taking a medication called "Provigil". It keeps you awake for exactly sixteen hours from the point of taking it. The military issue it to the troops during wars to prevent the troops from sleeping when they are under attack. It is an amazing medication and worked well for me. However, it does not make the original problems go away, it simply masks them. It also costs approximately $400 per month!

Needless to say, I was not looking for a tablet, I was looking for a cure!

I had developed red blotchy patches of skin on my buttocks. They were not painful or sore. I had noticed them in the mirror after showering one day. They were there for months. I saw many doctors about them and they did not know what would cause the blotches. Today, I suspect that it was the company cellphone electromagnetic emissions that were causing them, as I would keep the mobile phone in my back pocket. They cleared up after I left that company and I have never seen them since. The blotchy skin effect is commonly reported by people who have Electromagnetic Hypersensitivity.

During my development of the book "Toxic Electricity", I analyzed the environment that I was working in. I was working in a cubicle desk that was surrounded by other workers who had cellphones and wireless computer systems. My desk was very close to the electrical room that housed all of the computer network equipment for the building and the wireless router. The high voltage overhead utility power lines and poles in the street were approximately 30 feet from my desk! The airport was across the road and there would have been extensive RADAR and radio wave emissions from it. There may have been infra-sound and pollution issues as well. The company used radio frequency identification (RFID) controlled doors and I would pass through these perhaps 100 times per day to get between departments. I was also sitting near to the transmitting RFID door sensor of a very high traffic door, carrying a company smart phone and my own personal cell phone.

"The Bible is like a telescope. If a man looks through his telescope, then he sees worlds beyond; but, if he looks at his telescope, then he does not see anything but that."

Henry Ward Beecher

Florida

In 2009 I commissioned a very large utility solar power system over two months. It was an interesting experience that was setting the stage for finding the cure that I was looking for.

During the two months of commissioning, I had noticed some very strange behaviors in the people involved with the project. I was seeing aggressiveness, fatigue, and forgetfulness. I was also seeing habitual lying over commissioning issues that were showing up and that appeared to be caused by pressure for the project to be perceived as successful by the company management team. In conversations with the staff, they were telling me that they were not sleeping well and that they were having aches and pains throughout their bodies. Very similar conditions to my own!

One day, after spending the entire day working around the high voltage transformers, electronic power inverter systems and solar modules, I noticed that my smell was off. At the time, I was in the 24,000 volt switching center at the site and I could smell smoke when there was no smoke. The most amount of electrical power was in here, as it feeds into the electrical utility transmission system. It was a sunny day with approximately eighteen million watts of electronically generated harmonic electricity flowing through the room. There was approximately 10% harmonic distortion on the utility power sine wave.

I was absolutely convinced that something was on fire and the people that I was with were telling me that they could not smell it. I also appeared to be intoxicated. Later that day, I found that I could not stop drinking due to an insatiable thirst! I had been drinking during the day and I did not appear to be dehydrated, my urine was not dark, nor was I sunburned as I had sunscreen on, sunglasses, a wide brimmed hard hat, and a whole body arc flash suit. Everything appeared to be back to normal the next day.

During research for my books, I found that these symptoms are listed as Radio Wave Sickness (RWS). I was not surprised, as the power plant was producing excessive harmonics and nobody had warned me about the dangers of high powered electronic utility equipment that has excessive harmonic energy on it.

After leaving this project, I soon discovered that I could not remember computer passwords, phone numbers, alarm codes, and basic mathematics was difficult for me. It was clear that I had received a toxic brain exposure from the high powered electronic utility equipment. Nikola Tesla documents having a similar experience during his research and development.

"Every living being is an engine geared to the wheelwork of the universe. Though seemingly affected only by its immediate surrounding, the sphere of external influence extends to infinite distance."

Nikola Tesla

2010

I started to develop books on solar power systems and that led to the discovery of the "Multiple-Sun" effect. The multiple-Sun effect occurs anywhere that there are solar reflections taking place. Solar power systems with their reflective glass surfaces create it. I knew the effect was important and I started to develop it further. I found that it also occurs in city environments where there are large amounts of glass in buildings. It is particularly bad around glass covered tower buildings.

The multiple-Sun effect significantly raises the radiation levels in the human environment to above the radiation levels of Space. Bingo! I had discovered that I had developed radiation sickness over the years of extended exposure to radiation sources.

I also stopped taking the medications. I had been taking Provigil for the daytime and over the counter sleeping tablets to counteract the insomnia symptoms. This over the counter sleep medication was a range of melatonin, diphenhydramine and doxylamine succinate. The doctor has prescribed Seroquel, but I found that it made me feel really bad for the first hour in the morning.

The interesting thing is, it is commonly reported in the USA that approximately 50% of the population is taking prescription medications! I had noticed on my travels that many people that I have worked with are routinely taking medications. I was not alone in this lifestyle that had developed over the years. Unfortunately, many USA children are also in the same situation.

Within days I went into really severe drugs withdrawal. I literally could not get out of bed for a few days as I felt so bad. Flu like symptoms followed by really bad headaches for about two weeks that would not respond to medication. I had never experienced this before!

It slowly cleared up which led me to the understanding that if you take medications long term, then your mind and body will go toxic. The interesting thing was, my thought patterns changed! A calm mind replaced a mind that was constantly active with various thoughts. My insomnia also slowly cleared up. As such, it is better to avoid the medications if you can.

After doing the work with the development of the multiple-Sun effect in 2010, I knew that it was wise to balance it out and to spend a corresponding amount of time out of the Sun. For six months, I avoided sunlight. A few weeks into this process, I got extremely ill with flu like symptoms. My heartbeat was fluctuating and I had intense pains throughout my body. It was so bad that I thought that I was going to die! It lasted a few days and then slowly got better. It was clear at this point that I was in radiation withdrawal. About a month into the withdrawal I had my blood tested and everything was showing normal levels.

Extreme fatigue followed for a few months and that eventually cleared up. I noticed several weeks into the withdrawal process that my body was reacting to sunlight exposure, if I spent time outside in the sunlight, then I would have a big headache the next day.

I went to view Niagara falls with my friends and we rode right up to the bright white wall of water on the Maid of the Mist. For me, it was like drinking several beers, it made me develop symptoms of intoxication!

As time went by, my pains started to subside. Eventually, they disappeared! Today, after years of random aches and pains, I am pain free.

"The radiation detoxification process exists in nature. It is called: Hibernation."

Steven Magee

2011

After several months of avoiding the Sun, I had my blood tested again and it had gone low in both vitamin B12 and vitamin D. My diet had not changed, the only thing that had changed was my sunlight exposure. The vitamin D deficiency was expected, as it is well documented as being a photosynthesis vitamin. There was plenty of meat and fish in my diet for sources of B12, so being low on B12 was a surprise. So I concluded that the B12 deficiency was related to the lack of Sun exposure.

It is interesting to note that in Autistic children, vitamin B12 injections have been shown to significantly reduce their symptoms. I do currently believe that both Autism and Attention Deficit Disorder (ADD) are electromagnetic diseases.

I started to get 15 minutes of Sun per day, which is the current guidelines for maintaining adequate vitamin D levels. Much to my surprise, I eventually got to a period where extreme fatigue showed up and all that I wanted to do was sleep every day. My vitamin D and B12 levels appeared to continue to decline and had brought on the symptoms of Seasonal Affective Disorder (SAD). I increased the sunlight exposure time to an hour per day in the shade and that eventually fixed it.

Just for curiosity, I started to sunbathe and found that at two hours per day, the aches and pains came back. They were fixed by staying out of the Sun for a few days. I eventually established that my outdoor solar radiation levels are at 1 hour per day in the shade in sunny Arizona to maintain good health. My genetics are a mix of Irish and English with relatively white skin. My skin today is a golden brown. If you have darker skin, then your daily requirements for solar radiation exposure will be higher due to the pigmentation. I later realized that the aches and pains may have been caused by the high wireless radiation levels outside, as my plants were showing deformities in that area. Some parts of my garden have wireless radiation levels of approximately 700 millivolts per meter, which is considered very high by most electromagnetic radiation researchers. In the National Park forest, the wireless energy meter reads zero.

At this point, the main problem that I was showing was occasional fatigue. It was the kind of fatigue that makes you want to take a nap in the middle of the day. During research for the book "Toxic Electricity" I had realized that people who report Electromagnetic Hypersensitivity generally report fatigue. I started to research my human body voltage and found that there was a large AC waveform riding on my body. Turning off my home electrical circuits eliminated it. I also discovered that my tiled flooring in the home was electrified with "Stray Voltage" from the electrical utility neutral and started to wear slippers when home to prevent coming into contact with it. I changed all of my light bulbs from compact florescent lights (CFL) to conventional filament lights. I tested the CFL's and found that they had unnatural spectrums of light and radio wave emissions. I switched over to a diet rich in organic fresh fruit and vegetables and turned off the cell phone. These actions brought up my energy levels.

I should mention that due to my knowledge of how utility power companies willfully mislead the public, during the Fukushima nuclear disaster I changed my diet over to dried and canned food in March 2011 to avoid the surge of radiation contaminated food in the USA food system. During the following nine months, I noticed that my skin started to develop problems on my elbows with rough, dry and brittle skin. My teeth started to decay, and I was getting indigestion and stomach problems. Heart burn and acid reflux was an issue and I was constantly taking antacids to alleviate the symptoms. These problems fixed themselves after a few months of eating fresh organic food.

I concluded that extended exposure to preserved food is harmful to human health and the health problems can be simply fixed by eating fresh organic food.

I had noticed that the occasional fatigue completely cleared up when I went camping in remote National Parks, which I would do at least once per year. To clear the occasional fatigue up, I suspected that I was going to have to move to a different area, due to the high radiation levels around my property from the three cell phone towers that are approximately 2,000 feet to 2,300 feet from my home. I had planted trees and plants around my property when I purchased it and I knew that they would eventually reduce the radio frequency radiation levels by absorbing it.

"Only a full spectrum of natural light could promote full health in plants, animals, and humans."

Dr. John Nash Ott

2012

Watching the plants grow over the years led me to the understanding that things were not growing correctly in the garden. The extensive indoor plant experiments that I was performing showed me that the electromagnetic radiation environment of the entire home was extremely unnatural, as even my control plants were deforming! I had many Dieffenbachia (Dumb Cane) plants in the home and every one was deformed! There were zones around the outside of the home that were showing stress and growth problems in the plants. These were the entire west side of the home and the entire north east side of the home where the utility electrical equipment was located. The northwest part of the garden was the worst and there were areas that I had noticed that the plants would die when placed there. It did not matter what type of plant I planted in these locations, they would die after several months.

I took all of my wireless devices out of service in summertime 2012 and had the electrical utility company change out the automatic meter reader (AMR) for a conventional mechanical electric meter on both my home and the neighbors home. This appears to have cured some of the growth problems that I was seeing in my plants. It was clear that the utility company and my wireless devices had inadvertently turned my home and garden area into the equivalent of an antenna park! It improved the occasional fatigue, but did not fully clear it up. I did get very sore and sensitive teeth in the weeks following removing the wireless products, as did my neighbors. It appeared to be a withdrawal symptom from the wireless radiation. In summertime 2013 I had the first ever fruits that the garden had produced from a peach and a pomegranate tree. It was obvious that the wireless radiation exposures had been causing these trees to abort their fruit development in the previous years.

Many people report problems with metal coil mattresses. I checked mine out and found that it was acting as an antenna system for AC electricity and radio waves! I changed out my metal coil mattress to a latex foam mattress to see if that would help. It improved my sleep, but did not appear to improve the occasional fatigue.

I developed "Rotational Sleeping" when I became aware that there are now biological hotspots of wireless radiation in homes today. The technique revolves around making sure that I do not sleep in the same position each night. The simplest form of the technique is to move the pillow to the opposite end of the bed from the previous night, so that I would rotate 180 degrees each night. I prefer to sleep in a four position rotation cycle and this works well in large beds. I follow this pattern in a large bed:

1. **Left side of bed.**
2. **Rotate 180 degrees.**
3. **Right side of bed.**
4. **Rotate 180 degrees.**

This means that if there is a biological hotspot where my head rests, then it will only be subjected to that hotspot one night in every four. I found that my quality of sleep and daytime energy levels improved after adopting rotational sleeping.

A useful technique for assessing the quality of the environment in my bedrooms was the "Goldilocks" test. I had four bedrooms and I spent a week sleeping in each bedroom to see how I felt. I was quite shocked at how different each bedroom was to sleep in! The worst by far was the front bedroom that was next to the street. The second worst was the rear bedroom that has a view of a cell phone tower approximately 2,300 feet away. The bedrooms that were in the middle of the home were the ones where I was waking up feeling the most refreshed and I now sleep in one of these bedrooms. These two middle bedrooms have the

lowest radio frequency (RF) power levels and there are areas in them that will read zero RF power.

I tried the "Earthing" health technique for two reasons. I wanted to assess it for my book "Toxic Electricity" and I thought that it may clear up the fatigue. I saw my back tingle for about a week in the area where I was in contact with the earthing cable, so it definitely was doing something. However, as time went on I got the most severe bad back that I have ever had. It was in the base of my spine and badly affected my walking! It took a few weeks to clear up. Then I went into the worst period of heart arrhythmia that I have ever experienced! Fearing a heart attack, I decided to stop the technique. I tested the cable and found that it was acting as an antenna system and had a wide range of frequencies on it! The grounding cable health technique did not work for me, but there are people who say that it does work.

People had commented over the years that when they would enter my home that there was a strange odor. I had wondered for a long time where this odor was coming from, as I had noticed it myself from time to time. It was apparent when coming into the home after it had been locked up for several hours. I found that my kitchen island had an in-line sewer vent valve installed into it. These valves allow air to enter into the sewer system from the home and prevent the sewer gas from escaping. When the in-line vent valve ages, it may start to leak sewer gas. Replacing this fixed the odor problem. If you have one of these valves in your home, you should pay attention to it as sewer gas is explosive and poisonous!

I followed Dr. John Nash Ott's advice and installed ultraviolet (UV) transmitting plastic windows in the areas of my home where I spend my daytime. When compared to the crystal clear UV transmitting acrylic windows, my double glazed glass windows look green and dim! This heavily filtered colored light from the low-E double glazed glass windows appears to have been contributing to the fatigue issues that I was seeing. Using "Full Spectrum" glazing appears to have significantly reduced the occasional fatigue problem.

The health benefits that I observed during testing ultraviolet transmitting acrylic windows were:

- **Excellent daytime energy levels.**

- **Wonderful sleep cycle.**

- **Improved mental functioning.**

- **Brighter indoor environment.**

- **Indoor colors are vivid.**

- **The computer is more pleasant to work with. It appears to have significantly reduced the dry eyes and chapped lips that it gave me with long periods of use.**

- **Fruits ripen faster in the full spectrum light.**

- **Good health.**

In the first month that I installed this I did see some interesting aches and pains. My left ankle and my right elbow were aching for no reason whatsoever. I then got some intestinal pains that I have not had before. They cleared up after a few weeks and appeared to be due to the changes that were taking place in my body.

After the initial surge in health, I started getting the desire to occasionally nap again at lunchtime. I have established that I get full health whenever I go camping in remote National Parks or travel to areas that are rural with very low cell phone reception. While I have always associated good health with low cell phone reception, I do spend more time outside around nature on these trips.

I increased my outdoor time to two hours around solar noon in the shade. Generally I will read a book during this time. I will get a little direct sunlight exposure also, typically half an hour. This really brought up my energy levels.

This leads me to conclude that exposure to the peak in solar radiation that occurs around solar noon is essential to good health. My daily solar radiation exposure is to sit near to my shady ultraviolet transmitting full spectrum acrylic window while I develop my research and then to go out around solar noon for a couple of hours in the shade reading. I'll take a stroll around the garden in the direct sunlight during that time.

I moved my computer next to the shady ultraviolet transmitting window. When I work on it during the daytime, I now have the outdoors in my field of view. This enables my eyes, face and hands to get full spectrum daylight exposure all day long. My daytime light environment is now in tune with thousands of years of evolution. One could say that I have finally achieved resonance with the daylight environment!

"Mal-illumination is to light as malnutrition is to food."

Dr. John Nash Ott

2013

I discovered that the gas company installed a new version of their automatic meter reader (AMR) radiation transmitting device at my property. I do not know exactly when it was installed, but I asked around and it appears that it was installed sometime in January 2013. It was the reason why my health took a step back. The gas company installed them throughout the community, as I could see the same shiny AMR meters at other properties in the neighborhood. I tested it and it was emitting a radiation pulse every several seconds. The previous gas meter had no detectable radiation pulses coming from it. I started to watch my plants in that area to see if they would deform, go dormant or die.

To reduce the toxic effects of this, I moved my desk as far away from the AMR gas meters that I could in the home. It was the prudent thing to do. The World Health Organization class wireless transmitting devices as "Possibly Carcinogenic". There are no shortage of people who have traced their health problems to these devices and one can only wonder why they have not been banned. Moving further away from the AMR transmitters increased my energy levels which indicated that they were affecting my health. The symptoms that I observed were:

- January: Fatigue.

- February: Fatigue, waking up feeling hung over and lethargic.

- March: Fatigue, waking up feeling hung over and lethargic, fuzzy thinking and concentration problems.

- April: I abandoned my bed and started to sleep on the floor. I also increased the electromagnetic screening around the transmitting AMR meters. This reduced the severity of the symptoms.

I notified both the gas company and the Federal Communication Commission (FCC) that they were causing harmful biological interference at my property and to remove the AMR transmitting devices from the vicinity of my home.

In March 2013 I started to get really sick with classic Radio Wave Sickness symptoms. This is how the sickness progressed:

- Day 1 - Fuzzy thinking.

- Day 2 - Dizziness, fuzzy thinking, headaches.

- Day 3 - Dizziness, fuzzy thinking, headaches, insomnia.

- Day 4 & 5 - Dizziness, fuzzy thinking, headaches, insomnia, fatigue.

I had seen this range of symptoms appear with a similar rapid progression back in summertime 2012 when I went to stay in a mountaintop forest vacation area. When I researched the location from satellites I found that I had been staying approximately 1,000 feet from a large antenna park that had cell phone towers and multiple radome installations in it! The interesting thing was, my girlfriend showed a different rate of progression. She was symptom free until the fourth day when she started showing headaches, insomnia and fatigue. We were both relieved to leave that location and our symptoms rapidly subsided within hours of leaving the area.

It was clearly Radio Wave Sickness that had shown up, but what was causing it? My best guess was that I had moved into a hotspot of radiation and that it was affecting me. It was the correct assumption. I had been given a printer to repair and was using it daily to test it. I had noticed that it had built in Wi-Fi but was not using it. I tested the printer with my radio frequency meter and there was a large field of wireless radiation around it! I had been sitting just 2 feet away from the printer in a 1,000 mV/m radiation field daily and this was consistent with the symptoms that had shown up. It appears that wireless network printers exhibit a similar behavior to wireless network routers and continually fill the area with microwave radiation. It is for this reason that you should not sit near to devices like this. The best way is not to have wireless devices of any kind.

I had noticed that the ultraviolet acrylic windows were reacting to infra-sound. A pulse of energy would hit them and make them vibrate. It was very noticeable at my home and lasted less than a second. There was no wind present when I saw this occur. Out in the desert is a military bombing range that generates sonic booms. When I worked on Kitt Peak, I would hear the sonic booms frequently and they would shake the buildings! It appeared that I was detecting them at my home with my acrylic windows! This is concerning, as infra-sound is well known for its ability to make people sick.

In May 2013 I found that my toilets were electrified with stray voltage. When I would urinate into them this would make the drain wet and electrify them from the stray voltage in the street! I was curious and tested my showers and found that when the drain gets wet, it electrifies the shower! This is a concerning development, as it means that there are many toilets out there that are electrified with stray voltage. This is consistent with some trips that I took to the doctors several years ago with urethra problems that the doctor could not diagnose. I suspect that the stray voltage issue was much higher during that period. I only saw it for one year and then it spontaneously cleared up. Needless to say, now I know that my drains are electrified, I no longer urinate into my toilets. This action increased my energy levels. I did see quite severe headaches occur during the following two weeks that gradually subsided and this appeared to be a withdrawal reaction.

High activity muscle building exercise was a step that I had wanted to introduce for quite some time. I was reluctant to start doing it while I was dealing with and characterizing the earlier issues. I have always walked for exercise during this recovery process but I wanted to introduce a daily exercise regimen that made me really sweaty! Walking is not really exercise, as it does not work the entire body. This was evidenced by my weight increasing from 154 pounds in 2009 to

192 pounds in 2013. During that period I had led a sedentary life with most of my time spent at home. I started to follow a DVD workout routine every day. I lost 6 pounds in the first ten days! The thing that was very noticeable was that my hunger subsided and that I was content with smaller portions. My body shape change was noticeable as was my increase in muscle mass. After twenty days my weight had stabilized at 184 pounds and it was obvious that my fat was in the process of being converted into muscle, as the exercise routine had become enjoyable and my strength had significantly increased. By thirty days my stamina had developed and I was able to fully perform each exercise routine.

While I was setting up a structured water plant experiment, it caused me to investigate what exactly was in my drinking water filter. I had been advised by numerous people in Tucson to filter my water, as they believed that the drinking water was contaminated by industrial and mining activities in the area. I thought that I was carbon filtering my water. However, when I checked the water filter box, I found that there were ion exchange resin beads in addition to carbon. It appears that since 2007 that I was drinking carbon filtered ion exchanged water! I checked the filters out on the internet and sure enough, I found many complaints about them from people who had been made ill by using them. Naturally, I switched my drinking water back to standard faucet water from the utility company. Over the following weeks I saw my energy levels increase.

The gas company did eventually remove the biologically harmful AMR meter from my home. However, they refused to remove the one on the neighbors home just 15 feet away! I had actually requested that they remove four of their transmitting meters from within 100 feet of my bedrooms, but only the one on my home was changed for a non-transmitting meter. The gas company knows that these transmitting meters make me sick and are okay with that state of affairs. It is clearly a case of willful biological assault with known biologically harmful radio frequency devices that the military weaponized as they were so good at making the enemy sick! And it is happening at my home which represents my greatest financial investment! My home is not a place of safe refuge and this is a violation of the USA Declaration of Independence.

Heart arrhythmia and insomnia eventually showed up when I was sleeping on the floor. It was likely a combination of extended exposure to the transmitting utility meters in the area and the summertime stray voltage levels increasing on the concrete floor that I was sleeping on. This required a change in direction to seek good health.

The many plant experiments that I was performing with the Dieffenbachia plant had started to yield results that I had not expected. Some of the plants instead of extensively deforming were actually showing growth that was closer to the normal growth that the plants were displaying when I bought them. These experiments were:

- **Growing a Dieffenbachia with a battery powered wristwatch embedded in its roots.**

- **Growing a Dieffenbachia by watering it with hot tea that had cooled.**

- **Growing a Dieffenbachia by connecting a single cell 1.5 volt battery connected between the roots and the upper stem.**

- **Growing a Dieffenbachia by grounding the roots and soil to the conductive tiled floor. (Note: This only worked on the tiled floor furthest from the street and the utility electrical equipment.)**

So I started to wear the same model of resin strap battery powered analogue wristwatch, drink tea, connect myself to a 1.5 volt battery between the sole of my foot and wrist, and walk barefoot on the tiled floor furthest from the street.

Connecting to the 1.5 volt single cell battery caused me to develop very strong chemical smelling urine that was a similar odor to WD-40. The strong smelling urine had me concerned, so I stopped connecting to a battery and decided to instead turn my body into a battery! It is easily achieved

by ingesting electrolyte and metal supplements. A positive voltage of 0.5 volts at the finger relative to the grounded feet was developed using this process. This turned on the chemical smelling urine again. The urine chemical smell disappeared after a few months of taking the supplements and seemed to be a reaction to the 0.5 volts DC that had developed on the body.

It is clear from the many plant growth experiments that I have performed with the Dieffenbachia plant that an atmospheric DC voltage has gone missing in the modern world and this lack of DC atmospheric voltage is having far reaching consequences for all life where it is not present. It appears that a great biological price has been paid by the modern masses for the convenience of tall man-made structures, electricity and wireless radiation.

I was seeing poor digestion over the years that was marked by loose stools. I had become aware at this point that the extensive radio frequency fields that were passing through my home were interfering with the digestive system. This can be remedied by taking a digestive supplement. The most effective supplement that I identified was brewers yeast. I started taking a teaspoon dissolved in a glass of water with every meal. After a few months I found that I only needed one teaspoon daily. I also take a teaspoon of Psyllium Husk daily.

I had been wondering how much of the occasional fatigue was coming from the electrical transmitting utility meters. I got my answer in 2013 when we had a daytime power cut for several hours. The longer the power cut went on for, the bigger my headache became! It was clearly a withdrawal headache from the changed radiation environment, as the electrical meters stop broadcasting radiation when the power is off. There are no doubts that the electromagnetic interference that the electrical system generates is biologically harmful to the human.

Regarding the transmitting gas meters, I saw South West Gas take the manual meter reading at my home in December 2013 while I was out walking with my partner and our baby. A car stopped at our home and two men got out and went into the meter area. They came out and drove off. They were stopped for about two minutes. The car had a large antenna system on the roof and this is how they are currently obtaining the electronic meter readings. My community has both the old (Itron 40G) and the new style (Itron 100G) AMR/AMI gas meters. The old style appears to need to receive a signal from the car to start broadcasting, while the new type broadcasts pulsed radiation continuously. The car drove past us and we were about fifteen feet from the antenna system on its roof. I monitored our health after the AMR/AMI gas meter mobile transceiver car came through our area at lunchtime and I observed the following:

Day 1

- Skull pains that were off and on for a few hours.

- Headache appeared by 15:00 and lasted for a few hours before subsiding on its own.

- Extreme fatigue showed up at 17:00 and lasted a couple of hours. I was falling asleep while trying to have a conversation with a guest.

Day 2

- Woke up extremely thirsty.

- Headache developed during the morning that lasted all day.

- I became nauseous between 15:00 to 18:00.

- Intestinal pains in the evening.

- Thought patterns were off with some confusion and forgetfulness.

- Had to go to bed early due to an intolerable headache.

- Insomnia through the night.

- My three month old baby woke up two hours earlier than normal, was fussy, restless and refused to sleep more than half an hour at a time. Her behaviors were

41

distinctly different from her usual routine of sleeping for a couple of hours between feeds.

- Baby spitting up far more than usual.

Day 3

- My partner had to look after the baby as I had become so sick.

- Got out of bed at 12:00 with a severe headache that lasted all day.

- Hearing in both ears was showing issues that lasted all day. The sensitivity kept on changing.

- Baby woke up 2 hours earlier than normal.

- Baby spitting up far more than usual.

Day 4

- Headache all day long.

- Baby woke up 2 hours earlier than normal.

- Baby spitting up far more than usual.

Day 5

- Skull pains came back and were infrequent during the day.

- My partner was showing the Neurasthenia symptom of irritability.

- Baby woke up 2 hours earlier than normal.

- Baby screamed in pain for two hours and was inconsolable.

Day 6, 7 and 8

- Skull pains came back and were infrequent during the day.

The above appeared to be the biological reaction to the spike in radiation levels that occurred as all of the AMR transmitting meters in the area started to broadcast their radiation and to the gas company car radio frequency transmitter. I am wondering what radiation is being broadcast from that meter reading car to see such a severe set of reactions. I have not seen such a diverse and severe sickness for quite some time, so it was an unusual event for me. It may not have occurred had I been sitting inside the home as opposed to outside walking with the baby where the man-made radiation levels are much higher. I would suggest that if you see the utility meter reading car in your area, that you should probably go indoors for the rest of the day in order to protect your health.

I am sure that you would agree that these are concerning effects from the simple action of having gas meters read by the gas company! My partner had the same exposures and showed much milder effects as she is about three times less sensitive to radiation exposures than I am. She does not have any metal dental bridges that act as a "Dipole Antenna" system that I have. I am very concerned that my three month old daughter had this exposure to her ovaries and this may have an impact on her fertility later in life. We will find out in about four decades from now what her lasting effects are to this exposure. This was clearly a case of electronic assault by the gas utility company on my family.

The Tucson utilities Itron AMR/AMI radiation transmitting metering system is by far the most toxic transmitting system that I have come across in three years of biological radio frequency research. It is orders of magnitude more toxic than anything else that I have encountered. I have walked right up to the forest of high powered transmitters in the antenna park on Sandia Peak in Alberqueque, New Mexico, and have not seen reactions anything like this. The radiation levels are so high next to that antenna park that there are posted warnings in the car park! It is probable that many people are adversely reacting to the utility transmitting meter reading car and have not yet associated their sickness that occurs to the biologically harmful exposure. They are likely getting approximately a

week of sickness every time it passes through their neighborhood.

"Lyon, France, May 31, 2011 -- The WHO/International Agency for Research on Cancer (IARC) has classified radiofrequency electromagnetic fields as possibly carcinogenic to humans (Group 2B), based on an increased risk for glioma, a malignant type of brain cancer, associated with wireless phone use."

World Health Organization

2014

During a conversation in 2014 with my partner, she informed me that she had seen an improvement in health during the time that she had been living at my home. At her previous residence she had a high voltage power pole and power lines at the front and a utility electrical transformer at the back. She was also sleeping next to the fuse board and it had two radio frequency transmitting meters due to her solar power system. Her home was small on a tiny plot of land in a dense solar powered community near to downtown Tucson and an industrial area. She said that after she moved in with me that her degrading allergies that the doctor wanted to give her a prescription for miraculously cleared up! Curiously, someone had been cutting the grounding wires on several of the power poles and this is a common response to the problem of stray voltage and ground currents.

The occasional afternoon fatigue and high pitched "Microwave Hearing" buzzing ears were the only regular health symptoms that I was displaying by January 2014, along with the damage to my memory that occurred in 2009 at the high powered solar photovoltaic utility power plant. The fatigue was mild and tends to occur around noon and disappears by the evening. I was wondering if it was following the solar radiation power levels, as I was only seeing it appear when it peaks at solar noon. Solar noon appeared to trigger the fatigue and sunset eliminated it. It was an interesting phenomenon that appears to be tied to the peak in daily radiation levels! Wireless radiation induced fatigue is documented in the book "Insomnia, Fatigue and Cell Phone Towers" by Conrad LeBeau. In 1932, the German doctor Erwin Schliephake appears to be the first person in history to document the condition of Radio Wave Sickness, with fatigue being the primary feature of the sickness.

In January 2014 I started to read books out loud. I had been experimenting with Schumann resonances in 2013 and had not noticed any difference in energy levels. Reading out loud provided a way of resonating the body cavities. I progressed into the "Ohm" and "A-U-M" chanting to explore this area of body cavity resonance further. It strengthened my vocal cords and made public speaking far easier. I concluded that lack of vocal cord exercise was one of the problems for my poor ability in public speaking. My public speaking had been particularly affected from the point where I worked at the MDM Observatory and was sitting next to an electrical room daily. It got so bad that about a year after starting working there, I could not participate effectively in management meetings. I would get extremely anxious with very tight vocal cords that would hamper my ability to talk.

I started cutting my tree down in January 2014 that was outside of my front bedroom. I had identified that people who slept in the front bedroom got poor quality sleep and had linked to it the electromagnetic emissions of the tree. Testing had shown that the tree was planted in an area of stray voltage/currents/frequencies and that the top of the tree was in a 850 mV/m radio frequency field. I was only in contact with the tree for about an hour, but it brought on the Radio Wave Sickness symptoms of diarrhea, intestinal pains, insomnia and headaches in the few days that followed. I researched trees and found that they have been known to be filled with electrical energy for over a century! The radio frequency energy on a tree peaks at two thirds of its height and this was exactly where I was working in it. The headaches were continuous and would not clear up, so I started to take aspirin in February 2014.

I took one 325mg aspirin tablet daily for a week. This brought on heart arrhythmia for a couple of days. I then ramped up to 2 aspirin tablets every four hours. This brought on sneezing, sore eyes, runny nose and feeling run down. It cleared up my headaches, but my bones began aching. After 4 days, I became very fatigued, developed headaches and slept most of the day. I stopped taking the 650mg dosing after six days and reduced the dosing to 325mg every four hours. This cleared up the adverse symptoms and I continued this dose for one week. I then ramped down the aspirin over a week to the maintenance dose of 1 tablet daily of 325mg. As my body adjusted to the maintenance dose, I saw fatigue, disturbed sleep, strange dreams, lethargic in the morning and headaches. After four days at the maintenance dose, I developed chapped lips and a sore throat that lasted a few days. A few weeks later, I changed out the aspirin for an Alka-Seltzer tablet that contains 325mg of aspirin. This was due to wanting to introduce the sodium bicarbonate supplement that Alka-Seltza contains.

What appeared to happen was that the radio frequency exposure from the tree had caused rouleaux formations to occur in my blood which had caused clots in my brain to form. These clots did not dissipate after the radio frequency exposure was removed. The high dosing of aspirin acted like a blood thinner and dissolved the clots in my brain. I call dosing of aspirin that clears radio frequency induced clots:

Rouleaux Flushing

Rouleaux formations are a form of blood thickening and coagulation. I believe that it is a natural process that is designed to clot blood that reaches the surface of the skin. It appears that the "Skin Effect" of high frequencies traveling predominantly at the surface layer is a factor in the healing of wounds. If the radio frequency is sufficiently powerful, then it triggers rouleaux formations to start occurring deeper in the blood system of the body. This is an unnatural state and should be avoided for good health.

One of the avoidance effects that I now recommend is to keep trees and plants short in areas of stray voltage/currents/frequencies and high powered radio frequency fields. Plants and trees should be just a foot or so tall in areas of stray voltage/currents/frequencies. Trees should be no higher than the roofs of the homes in areas that radio frequency transmitters are installed into.

It is interesting to note that heart defibrillators are now being installed into schools, as children appear to be having heart attacks. Perhaps this is related to the rouleaux formations now that children are in classrooms that are filled with dirty electricity from electronic products and wireless radiation from computer Wi-Fi networks and laptop computers?

In February 2014, I started to boil my drinking water. I had been performing an experiment regarding different types of water and had discovered that the Tucson water plant was showing some of the most stress. I had become aware that water can be structured by magnetic field exposure and radio frequencies. I was also aware that the structuring could be undone by boiling the water. I had been attending cell phone tower hearings and had noted that Tucson Water was allowing applications for cell phone towers on its water pumping and storage sites throughout Tucson. I knew that it was likely that the water had been exposed to radio frequencies and the magnetic fields of pumping equipment prior to arriving at my home and may have had significant unnatural structuring to it.

Caring for my five month old daughter had prevented me from keeping up the daily exercise regimen that I had been following. As such, I was looking for an alternative form of exercise that would not wake up a sleeping baby. It turned out that standing all day is actually a form of exercise that burns calories and keeps the body in tension. I rearranged my computer into a standing desk and started to stand while working on it. It was an excellent form of exercise that requires minimal effort. I tend to sway from side to side when standing up to increase the calorie burning. I combined it with walking the baby every day.

In March 2014 I started to walk barefoot on my tiled floors. I considered the floors to be relatively safe outside of air conditioning season, where the high loads of the air conditioners cause significant levels of stray voltage to occur. Unfortunately, it seemed to cause insomnia and disturbed sleep patterns. As I continued to walk barefoot inside the home, I found that the skin on my feet became brittle and started to develop cracks that were raw and very sore. I was getting aches and pains in my feet during the night. Walking became painful, so I stopped the technique and let my feet heal. A headache developed during the following two days that appeared to be a withdrawal reaction. I had previously tested my floor and found that the Dieffenbachia plant would deform on the front hallway and kitchen floors. It grew well on my master bathroom floor. I moved my standing desk into the bathroom and tried it again. This time it worked with no adverse feet effects! It matched what I had seen in the master bathroom Dieffenbachia plant. However, as time went on I started to see heart arrhythmia and sore knees and by the end of April 2014 I stopped using the Earthing health technique.

By March 2014 I had established that the occasional afternoon fatigue that I was observing was occurring in every room of the home. I had moved my standing desk around the home and had set it up in the living room, master bathroom and the center bedroom of the home and I could not detect any difference between them. However, when I would work outside for the day, it would not show up. This indicated that it was not being caused by a wireless device, but rather by some problem inside of the home itself. This was a strong indication that the home wiring was emitting some kind of strange electromagnetic radiation. I tested my home wiring over several days and found:

- The harmonics were varying during the day.
- The level of electrical noise was high on the wiring.
- The wiring was acting like an antenna system.

I reconnected my ground rods in March 2014 that I had previously disconnected, as they were making the stray voltage worse around the property. I had done enough research by this point to realize that the two 8 foot long ground rods would alter the radio frequency content of the home wiring. I watched my health and did not see any improvement in it during the following week.

My next step was to install large capacitors at the fuse board to see if they would alter the emissions from the home wiring. Large capacitors have three definite functions on the AC electrical system:

* They act like short circuits to high frequencies.
* They store energy.
* They create reactive current flow.

Small capacitors of 0.1 microfarad and below do not have the ability to store significant energy. I had previously installed a capacitive filter on the home that was made up of capacitors of 0.1 microfarad and below. The large capacitors were added to see if they would alter the electrical system by providing this storage function. Large capacitors are generally referred to as "Smoothing Capacitors", as they have the ability to absorb spikes in energy and frequencies. The more distortion and electrical noise that is on the system, the bigger the capacitors have to be. I started with 47.5 microfarad capacitors connected between live1 to neutral, live2 to neutral and live1 to live2, giving a total of 142.5 microfarads. Each week I would add three more capacitors to the electrical system. I did not notice any significant change in health in the initial few weeks of doing this.

It is reported that many people have improved their health by adding large capacitors to their electrical system. I have encountered numerous people in my research who say that they have worked in reducing sickness and fatigue in their clients. However, I have also encountered some people who say that they made their conditions worse or saw no improvement. There are no doubts that installing large capacitors changes the characteristics of the home electrical system and it is a good way to investigate clearing up EHS for some people. The two leading capacitive filers available in the USA are:

* STETZERiZER filters.
* Greenwave filters.

Both are offered with money back guarantees if you feel that they did not work for you. I purchased "Motor Run" capacitors from an air conditioning wholesaler and made my own capacitive filters. It was cheaper to do so. However, for the general public, the commercial filters are a comparable cost; especially so when you factor in the packaging and assembly that the manufacturer had to do and note that there is no need to employ an electrician, as they simply plug into your existing electrical outlets. AC motor run capacitors are an expensive product and you should factor in several hundred dollars to install sufficiently high capacitance on your electrical system to reduce the biologically harmful dirty electricity effects.

The Stetzerizer filter appears to be based on a 20 microfarad capacitor and their powerstrip appears to use a 40 microfarad capacitor. Greenwave filters have three different models:

- Spectrum 2500 – three capacitors, including high and low frequency mitigation – more than 25 microfarad.

- Spectrum 2400 – seven capacitors with super broadband frequency coverage – more than 24 microfarad.

- Broadband 1500 – extremely wideband range – 5 capacitors totalling 15 microfarad.

Both manufacturers claim health improvements and this is supported by the findings of independent electromagnetic radiation researchers. Greenwave states *"we have over 500 testimonials of improvement in health, thinking, cognitive abilities, energy, focus, clarity, reduced myalgia, less headaches, less need for asthma inhalers, lower blood sugar for diabetics, etc.".* Most published research has been done with the Stetzerizer filter and this reflects that it was the original capacitive filter. People that research dirty electricity health effects use their "Microsurge Meter" and it has become the standard for electromagnetic researchers.

I did encounter some adverse health effects while researching capacitive filters:

- **My partner was showing fatigue, muscle aches and driving errors after I installed a 47.5 microfarad capacitive filter in her bedroom. I tested the master bedroom for magnetic fields and found that it was filled with them. The wiring for the bedroom had a wiring error that the capacitive current flow was causing magnetic fields. Removing the capacitor cured the problems.**

- **The same capacitor was installed in the living room. The next day I had a headache, was fatigued and feeling sick. My 7 month old daughter woke up crying, was irritable and vomited, which was very unusual. Both beds that we slept in were about 18 feet from where the capacitor was located. Some people do report that filtering capacitors make them sick and this experience matched those reports. I removed the capacitor from that location. I tested the capacitors and found that they were emitting radio waves. The electrical circuit also had a wiring error. It took several days for us to recover from the biologically harmful exposure and it was a clear warning for me not to perform electrical experiments in the vicinity of the nursery.**

After seeing these negative health effects, I sent out two questions to the EHS forum. The first was what negative health problems had been seen with capacitive filters and the second was what health improvements had been seen with them. No one responded to the improved health question, although a person contacted me privately from the forum to say they know people who have had their health improved by them. One person responded to the negative health question, stating that they gave him headaches and he had removed them. Two other people contacted me privately and stated that they were made sick by them and they had also removed them. It appears to be critical where to place these filters in the home and you should be wary of installing them near to sleeping areas and next to where people spend their daytime due to the electromagnetic interference emissions from them. Some homes appear not to be suitable for the installation of these and it is probably related to:

- How the homes were wired.

- The construction type of the home.

- The electrical products in the home.

- The electrical grounding system of the home.

- The levels of dirty electricity being supplied by the electrical utility.

- High rise buildings where the apartment is far from the electrical ground rods.

- Dense apartment complexes, due to the extensive dirty electricity effects of many people's electronic products on the electrical system.

I do not recommend installation of large microfarad capacitive filters without using a magnetic field meter. Installing these onto circuits that have wiring errors may fill the room with magnetic fields. I recommend that before and after magnetic field readings be performed when installing them to avoid the adverse health effects that magnetic field exposure may create. Electrical wiring errors that create magnetic fields are common.

Testing of the home electrical grounding system did show that installing capacitors changes the stray voltage and frequency content of it. My conclusion was that it is best to stay around 400 microfarad of capacitance on the system which is what the manufacturers recommend. I took my capacitive system to over 800 microfarad and found that too much capacitance appears to have the ability to make you sick.

I did not notice any change in my electrical utility bill during the period that I tested the capacitors. I eventually removed the large capacitors, as I did not observe any improved health, only negative health outcomes. They appeared unsuitable for use at my home.

Based on my research, you should be aware that a near exposure to a large microfarad capacitor connected to your electrical system may be a biohazard. Places where you find large microfarad capacitors in the home and workplace are:

- **Air conditioning systems.**

- **Central heating systems.**

- **Appliances that have motors, such as dishwashers, washing machines, dryers, refrigerators, fans and so on.**

- **Gas discharge lights that have conventional magnetic ballasts, such as florescent lights, sodium lights (street lights), mercury vapor lights (street lights), and so on.**

- **Power factor corrector (PFC) systems.**

You should avoid being near to these when they are operating due to the possible electromagnetic radiation emissions from their large microfarad capacitors and associated wiring.

By April 2014 I had completed cutting the tree down and all that was left was the main trunk. It had taken several weeks to do, cutting down just one trash can full per week. To my surprise, I had seen extensive biological reactions in the plants in the area by the time it had gone:

- A Cats Claw vine that had shown extensive stress for many years burst into life. It initially showed more stress in the first few weeks of cutting the tree down by showing very small leaves on the new growth. By the time the tree was cut down, this growth had returned to the normal rates of growth for this variety of vine. This leads me to ponder if there is an optimum size for the tree where the biologically harmful electromagnetic fields that it radiates peak?

- The Cats Claw vines on the front of the home were growing at a much slower rate than the same vines elsewhere. The growth rates drastically increased, as did the leaf size.

- The healthy Palo Verde tree next to it started showing stress and had died by the time the tree was cut down.

- The Sage Bush next to the tree was healthy at the start of cutting down the tree but was showing stresses by the time I had finished. Parts of the bush had gone brown and appeared dead.

- My health improved after cutting down the tree. I was showing far less daytime fatigue.

Having seen the results of cutting down this tree, I started to cut down the large bush that was in the utility equipment area. The plants in that area had shown stress for years. Some were barely alive.

I found that taking one Alka Seltza tablet daily for a few months had started to affect my health. During this time I had a cold sore, which I had not seen for some years. I do have to query whether it was related to the high levels of sodium bicarbonate in my system reacting with sunlight exposure? Eventually, I was getting irritable and forgetful! I changed the dose from 1 Alka-seltza tablet daily to 1 tablet weekly. I went through withdrawal over the next few days that comprised of the allergy symptoms of a runny nose and sneezing, with some fatigue. I continued to dose with one 325 mg aspirin tablet daily.

I was researching the ancient native cures and I found that it was common in many cultures to eat clay. Research into birds also revealed that some species eat clay. I was particularly interested in the habits of birds as they fly in a high radiation environment and have to deal with the natural and man-made radiation exposures. I also discovered that the astronauts are thought to be eating clay while on board the International Space Station. By this time, my plant experiments were showing radio frequency treated

water to have similar characteristics to reverse osmosis and steam distilled water. These waters are mineral deficient and mineralization can be achieved with clay. I knew that my body was mostly water and was in radio fields, so it would be exhibiting similar characteristics to the radio frequency treated water. As such, I introduced edible clay into my diet in April 2014 to create mineralization in my body water. One teaspoon dissolved in water daily.

In May 2014 I unplugged my kitchen appliances:

• Dishwasher.

• Microwave & kitchen extractor fan.

• Gas cooker.

They all had electronic control panels and I was suspicious that they may be putting dirty electricity onto my home wiring. That night, both my partner and myself had very unusual buzzing in our ears and our baby was restless all night. We only saw a reaction to the appliances being unplugged for that night only. The following week, I put the refrigerator on a timer. You need to be careful about the timer that you use for your refrigerator, as it has a large motor that will exceed the electrical specifications of most timer switches. I used a Intermatic TN311 15 amp heavy duty grounded timer to control my refrigerator. I set it up so that it runs all day up until 23:00. It then turns off until 02:00. It runs again between 02:00 and 03:00. It turns off from 03:00 until 05:30, when my partner gets up and starts to make breakfast. I turned the thermostat to the coldest setting to offset for the refrigerator warming up slightly while it is off during the night.

I did not tell my partner that I had done this, as she was becoming adverse to my experimentation with the electrical system and human health. The refrigerator was breast milk central for our eight month old daughter and my partner viewed it like gold. Anything that could put our gold at risk would get me into trouble! I also unplugged the washer and dryer. The next day I woke up with far more energy and feeling very refreshed! It matched my findings that the most biologically harmful exposures occur to the human during sleep.

The refrigerator has a 15 microfarad capacitor in it that I suspect gives out biologically harmful electromagnetic interference when the motor runs. I should mention that my kitchen appliances were all stainless steel and that the stainless steel may be acting as flat plate radio transmitters for the electrical grounding system dirty electricity effects. I now recommend standard painted appliances for this reason, as painted appliances insulate the appliance metal from contact with the air and reduce the radio transmitter efficiency.

My partner found out a few days later that I had installed the timer and was really mad at me! Strangely, I could not help but laugh at her as she was expressing her anger at the situation. A little research into multivitamin toxicity revealed that the laughing effect is a sign of zinc overdosing. I was taking the recommended dose for the multivitamin of two capsules a day that made a dose of 30 mG of zinc, so it was a surprise to find that I was in the zinc overdose state. I had also noticed during this time that trips to the kitchen were becoming difficult, as I was putting things in the wrong places and then could not find them later. It was possible that I was also overdosed from other vitamins in the multivitamin. I dropped the multivitamin back to one capsule per day to rectify this. I did not see a withdrawal reaction to the reduced dosing.

Measuring the currents that the appliances were taking revealed that they were consuming electricity when plugged in:

- 0.09 amp - 120 volt microhood.

- 0.08 amp - 120 volt washing machine.

- 0.06 amp - 120 volt gas cooker.

- 0.04 amp - 120 volt dishwasher.

- 0.04 amp - 240 volt clothes dryer.

By consuming current in standby meant that they were also passively emitting electromagnetic interference

when not in use! I was not surprised. All appliances really should completely disconnect from the electrical system when not in use and this is easily effected by placing the outlet that they plug into in an accessible location so that they can be unplugged from the electrical system. It is preferable to disconnect appliances when not in use to prevent their metal cases from acting like antenna systems and filling your home with wireless radiation emissions from a dirty electrical grounding system. It also prevents ground loops from occurring, appliance failures and appliance fires.

I was becoming forgetful in general and in the kitchen I was putting things away in the wrong places. This was concerning, as I knew that these were signs of Dementia and Alzhiemer's disease. This had occurred after I was well into developing the supplementation techniques for Electromagnetic Hypersensitivity. My partner was also telling me that my personality had significantly changed. I decided to stop dosing daily with aspirin and to see what happened. Within a few days I had a headache for two days that was followed with a day of sneezing and a runny nose. When I worked at the W. M. Keck Observatory at approximately 13,796 feet, I was taking aspirin daily to offset the headaches that I would get from altitude sickness. It was likely that I had developed aspirin poisoning while working there from this habitual long term daily dosing of aspirin. I saw many of the other staff members doing the same thing! Reducing the vitamin and aspirin dosing resulted in the forgetfulness subsiding. Adverse side effects are something to be aware of when supplementing and you should ensure that you are aware of the adverse side effects that are known to show up.

Regarding Autism, many people notice the onset of Autism symptoms in their children at the age of two. Babies are usually sitting at the table eating foods at the age of one. For some of them, a year later the onset of Autism is evident. My experience with supplementation indicates that after approximately one year of supplementing, adverse brain symptoms show up and these are cleared by reducing the dosing levels of the supplements. Are some of these Autistic children simply taking too many supplements? This can

occur through eating too much vitamin fortified foods, taking vitamin supplements and medications.

During my research it had become apparent that I was getting strange health symptoms whenever there was solar flare or sunspot activity. I would typically show fatigue, insomnia and skull pains during these periods. Just to make sure that I was not alone in this observation, I would send out a post to the Electromagnetic Hypersensitivity forum asking if other people were reacting. Sure enough, I would get replies from people saying that they were having adverse reactions also. Solar activity greatly affects the ground level radiation environment and this can be sensed by electrically sensitive humans.

In May 2014 I troubleshooted the electrical circuit that was creating strange magnetic fields in the master bedroom. I found that the electrician had wired up the switched socket in the room incorrectly. The electrician had inadvertently created what is known as an "Induction Loop" on the neutral and live wires. This was creating the strange magnetic fields and inducing energy into everything in the room. I rewired the circuit correctly and inspected my other switched socket in the living room. The electrician had made the same error there also. Repairing these wiring errors removed the high magnetic fields. The day after repairing the master bedroom wiring error, we both had a feeling of sickness that was akin to car sickness. It was gone by the evening. Over the following weeks my energy levels increased. These common wiring errors and how to detect and repair them are documented in the excellent book "Tracing EMF's in Building Wiring and Grounding" by Karl Riley. He estimates that 60% to 80% of USA homes have wiring errors!

Reading Karl Riley's book made me realize that there may have been a ground loop occurring on my cable TV connection. My cable TV comes into the home at the garage and then goes out to the master bedroom where it is distributed around the home. I found that the cable TV wire was grounded in both locations to the home electrical ground. I disconnected the electrical ground from the cable TV wire in the master bedroom to prevent this.

On May 26th 2014, the majority of Tucson had a power cut. I had been waiting quite some time for this to occur, as I wanted to see how my grounding system looked when there was no power in my area. This is the reason why I recommend that people have battery powered test equipment, as you can still perform measurements when there is no utility power. I took a look at the electrical grounding system with my oscilloscope and found that the waveform was very different to what it was with the utility system energized. I took some measurements and video and established that the utility combined ground and neutral connection was approximately ten times lower when it was off. It was approximately 0.3 volts peak to peak when it was off and when it came back on it was approximately 3 volts peak to peak!

The utility visited my home in 2011 and produced fraudulent stray voltage readings. When I pointed this out to them and requested that they repeat the readings, they closed the case, leaving me with electrified floors, an electrified garden and electrified drains that were exceeding the allowable animal contact voltage of 0.5 volts RMS AC on the electrical grounding system. I reported this to the Arizona Corporation Commission who regulate the power company, but no response was ever received. I have noticed a similar trend with other complaints that I have filed to them.

I called the electric company the next day and in the afternoon a very strange man arrived at my home! He did not hand me a business card identifying himself as a utility company employee, as the other people had done so in the past. I asked him for his business card and his response was that he never had one. So I asked him to write down his information for my records and he refused. I asked him for his first name, he refused, so I asked him for his last name and he refused. So I had a strange mystery man from unknown origin who was apparently going to diagnose my stray voltage fault.

Needless to say, a bad situation got worse, he said he was leaving because I kept on asking for identification. My response was to go and grab my video camera to get some video of this mystery man to report him to the Police. The utility company had issued a warning at the time about fraudulent imposters and to be careful. So I started to video the strange man's truck with him sitting inside of it. He was on the phone at the time. After he saw that I had video of him, he appeared to change his mind and stayed. However, like in 2011, no measurements of stray voltage were performed. I instructed him to do it and offered to help him, but after he had inspected my utility meter, he was leaving. I called the utility company to establish his identity and they hung up on me! So I reported the incident to the Police and gave them a copy of the video of the mystery man. The next day I filed a complaint to the Arizona Corporation Commission and sent the video to the local media.

About a week later I saw a response from the electrical utility company to their government regulator that was largely an imaginative fantasy of events that had occurred at my property. It is important to realize that when dealing with utility companies, that they will engage in elaborate fantasies regarding their customers. I have seen at least two other utility companies engage in these fantasies. You know that when a utility company is going down the fantasy route, they are likely hiding some illegal activity that they are engaging in. Fabricating fictional stories to their government regulator is just one of the many illegal activities that they engage in.

Electrical utility companies know that if they can drag out a stray voltage complaint by not correctly performing the measurements and by blatantly denying that the condition is occurring at your home, that in a few months the actionable levels of stray voltage will disappear. At that point, there is nothing to repair and they know that you will have to wait several months more until the next air conditioning season to report it again and they will likely give you the same fools errand! Stray voltage is generally caused by undersized neutral cables or higher than normal impedance neutrals (corrosion and bad connections) on the utility system and shows up when everyone turns on their air conditioners in summertime. This causes a volt drop condition to occur on the neutral that shows up as a much higher than normal neutral voltage at the home. Unfortunately, because the neutral is also the ground in Tucson, it electrifies your grounded electrical equipment cases, your copper plumbing, your conductive floors, your garden, your trees, your swimming pool, the street, and anything that is electrically conductive that has a connection to it with biologically harmful electricity!

I had been researching the Earthing health technique and I knew that this stray voltage was biologically nasty! It has all kinds of strange frequencies in it that are much higher than the 60 Hertz utility frequency. I knew that barefoot contact with lower levels of it through the electrified flooring brought on sore knees, heart arryhthmia and would cause the skin on my feet to crack and become painfully sore. Contact with it through an antistatic wrist strap would make me sick after approximately a week. Sleeping in the room next to the electrified tree brought on strange dreams and chronic daytime fatigue. I was getting irritable in summertime. It had become an issue that I wanted repaired, as my daughter was now rolling all over the floors. What would the electromagnetic emissions do to her in the long term? The police, the electrical utility company, the water company, the Arizona Corporation Commission, the Arizona Attourney General, and the home owners association all know about this electrification of my home, garden and the street with stray voltage and I have yet to see a single measurement be performed by any of them that would show it.

Some of the mistakes that people engage in when they find that they have a stray voltage problem are:

- Installing lots of ground rods – This electrifies the ground around the property and increases the levels of stray currents passing through the ground. It may make you sicker.

- Installing a ground ring around the perimeter of the property – This causes electrification of the entire property and ground currents will radiate out from the ground ring. It may make you sicker.

Some of the things that do improve the situation seem to be:

- Stray voltage isolator – This isolates the high voltage grounding system of the utility transformer from the combined ground and neutral connection that the utility supplies to you. In the event of a fault condition it automatically connects the transformer high voltage grounding system to the combined ground and neutral connection that the utility supplies to you in order to clear the fault. When the fault clears, it isolates the home grounding system from the utility high voltage grounding system. This is something that your utility company has to do, and they are known to refuse to acknowledge stray voltage problems. You may need to take them to court to effect this.

- Passing current of the opposite phase down the electrified neutral connection – You can use the impedance of the utility neutral cable to create an opposing voltage that the utility is supplying to you. You may have to send 50 to 100 amps down the neutral cable to create this cancellation effect. It is easily achieved in air conditioning season by using multiple 120 volt air conditioning units that can be switched on or off on the correct phase as needed to pass cancellation current down the neutral.

- High frequency mitigation – The electrical utility system is heavily contaminated with high frequencies. These can be filtered off into the ground by using capacitive filters. You should keep your capacitive filters at the fuse board and have everything inside metal grounded conduits and boxes, as they will be emitting a wide range of strange frequencies that they are filtering from the utility system.

- Removing the home foundation grounding system – Many homes and offices have been built that use the concrete foundation as the electrical grounding system.

63

This is a bad idea that should be discontinued, as it electrifies the foundation that you walk on! Even wearing insulated shoes will not protect you, as the foundation will be emitting electromagnetic fields that will couple into your body. The entire foundation is generally electrified with this system, which is commonly called an "Ufer ground" in the industry. The solution is to disconnect the home foundation electrical ground connection and to install electrical ground rods away from the home foundation. You should insulate the electrical grounding cable that goes out to the ground rods by running it through plastic conduit.

- Disconnection of ground rods – Some ground rods are known to electrify the surface ground with voltage for about 100 feet in radius. Disconnection of the electrical ground rods does not meet the electrical codes of the USA and may increase the probability of electrical damage during electrical faults. However, it does reduce the electrification of the ground and reduces ground currents. You would be liable for any problems that may result from this action.

- Move the electrical meter and the ground rods out to the street – This will reduce the effects of radio frequency transmissions from the utility meter and grounding system electrification effects on the home foundation.

I upgraded my electrical grounding system after much research on the subject. My home was using the Ufer ground which uses the home concrete foundation and I found that it was electrifying the floors of the home. To prevent this, I changed my grounding system to the following:

- Ground rod 1: 6 feet from home foundation and electrical fuse board, driven 18 inches below the surface. Copper underground cable connection from the fuse board to the ground rod insulated in PVC pipe. The PVC pipe insulates the surface soil from the bare copper ground conductor and reduces the stray voltage electrification effect.

- Ground rod 2: At least 6 feet from the home and at least 6 feet towards the street from ground rod 1, driven 18 inches below surface. Connected to ground rod 1 through insulated PVC pipe with copper cable.

- Both ground rods had low growing plants above them on irrigation to improve the ground connection and lower the electrical impedance.

- Disconnection of the concrete foundation electrical ground to avoid lightning damage to the home foundation (cracked foundation) and electrification of it (stray voltage/currents/frequencies).

- I plan on installing a 3/4" high frequency ground hollow copper pipe (standard 3/4" copper plumbing pipe) from the fuse board to ground rod 1. Run next to the existing ground cable to prevent creating a ground loop and inside of PVC pipe to insulate it. The last 1 foot of the copper pipe that is connected to the ground rod should not be insulated to give it a good ground connection to dissipate the high frequencies. (Note: You will not find this in the National Electric Code; radio operators and lightning conductors use copper ground pipes).

The building foundation ground (commonly called an Ufer) can be biologically hazardous. The premise of the building foundation grounding system is that all of the steel in the foundation is welded together and is electrically conductive. A copper wire is welded to the foundation metalwork to connect the electrical system to this metal grid. This copper wire is connected to the fuse board neutral and it passes whatever voltages, currents and frequencies it likes into the home foundation. Some home foundations are radiating electromagnetic energy from them and the people in these homes are likely sick and possibly diseased. You probably would not want to be inside an Ufer grounded home during a lightning strike to the home, as a very high voltage may appear throughout the home foundation. **If you happened to be stepping from the inside of the home to the outdoors during the lightning strike, you may be electrocuted! For biological purposes, the Ufer ground is to be avoided. Unfortunately in Tucson, a high lightning city, it is extensively used in new home construction.**

You need to be careful about having your electrical grounding system too far away from the fuse board, as it may become high impedance to high frequencies. A high impedance ground to frequencies is called an "Unground" in the radio industry and it causes havoc with their radio equipment. A hollow copper pipe is best to use for the high frequency ground, as high frequencies like to travel down the outside of a conductor and not the center of it. This is called the "Skin Effect".

While researching ground loops, I learned that some appliances connect the electrical ground to the neutral. This creates a ground loop that may make people sick. Appliances can also have metal feet and those that do typically create a ground loop through the conductive floor that they are in contact with. The ground loop from the metal feet is easily broken by placing plastic insulators under the feet. The internal electrical ground to neutral connection is easily broken by unplugging the appliance when not in use. I unplugged all of my appliances and the only appliance that was left connected when not in use was the refrigerator, for obvious reasons.

In June 2014, we went to stay in a hotel in Venice Beach, California. I knew the hotel had Wi-Fi and was not looking forward to the exposure. My worst fears were met when we found our room. Right outside was the wireless router! I was going to request a change of room, but decided to use the experience as a test to see how sensitive I was to Wi-Fi radiation. We stayed in the hotel for three days and two nights. Much to my surprise I saw no reactions whatsoever to the Wi-Fi. Nor to the high radiation environment of Venice Beach. It appeared that the last year of work that I had put into making the human mind and body resistant to wireless radiation emissions had paid off! We stayed at friends homes that had Wi-Fi and also saw no reactions to it.

In July 2014 I decided to have my root canal removed. There were a few reasons that made me decide to do this:

- The root canal was first done in Spain in 2000 and was very painful from time to time when I would bite on something.

- It was redone in Hawaii in 2004 and showed the same problems afterwords. I just put up with the pain the second time.

- I was concerned that the pain that I was having was a sign of something more serious.

- I could sense what appeared to be a DC voltage every time I touched it with my tongue.

- I knew that it had a metal cap and that metal acts as an antenna system and increases wireless radiation exposures in the human.

- Research into trees had shown that trees slowly die when too much metal (typically nails) is placed into them. I suspected that the same thing may be occurring in the human. As such, I wanted to reduce the amount of metal implants in my body to just my two metal dental bridges.

- The bad reaction that I had displayed to the Southwest Gas radio frequency meter reading car was concerning and I wanted to reduce the amount of metal implants to prevent such a severe reaction from occurring to a close exposure to a biologically toxic transmitter system.

I had it X-rayed and found that the root was fractured. Apparently, when the root is fractured, the only solution is removal. This is what should have happened in Hawaii back in 2004, instead of it being redone. The extraction went well and I was very relieved by what I saw come out of the root canal – a metal rod! I did not know it

was even there, it is apparently common to find metal rods supporting the metal cap on the root canal. They appeared to be made out of dissimilar metals and may have been creating a battery effect within my mouth. They were most likely acting as a "Dipole Antenna" system. In high electromagnetic fields, there may have been arcing occurring between them that would create radio wave emissions, similar to what occurs on high voltage power pole metal work.

I did not have much of a reaction to having it removed during the first 24 hours, however, the next three days were marked by a very large headache that would not respond to medication. It was painful to move my head, as it would make the headache even worse! I mostly stayed in bed during this time while what appeared to be withdrawal effects cleared out of my system. The gum healed up within two weeks and I was relieved that I had made the right decision to have it removed as it appeared to have been releasing toxins into my system.

Root canals have a bad reputation in the natural medicine field and you should consider having them removed if you are showing health issues. It appears to be mixed as to whether the health of people improves or not after the removal. One thing for sure, you are removing what is a decaying dead piece of the human body from your system.

During performing radio frequency measurements at my home in August 2014, I noticed that there was a pulsing spike of radiation in the master bedroom. I traced it to my partners Apple iTouch. The strange thing was, we knew that this device was emitting a pulse of radio frequency approximately every 45 seconds and had put it into airplane mode to stop it. We had not tested it afterwords, as we had assumed that airplane mode disabled all emissions from it. However, that was not the case! The device was clearly showing an airplane on its display. I checked the settings and airplane mode was on, as was Wi-Fi. I turned the Wi-Fi off and this stopped the pulses of radiation that it was emitting. It was a lesson that airplane mode should not be relied upon to disable wireless transmissions from a device and that you should also disable the wireless transmitter.

After extensive lifestyle changes that had yielded greatly improved health, I was still struggling to clear up the afternoon fatigue. I decided to revisit an earlier aspect of my research. I had noticed during research for the book "Toxic Light" that I would get insomnia if I looked up to the blue sky for an extended period. I got to wondering if I did this daily if the insomnia would subside and be replaced with all day energy? I knew that people were using light boxes that used high intensity blue light to treat Seasonal Affective Disorder (SAD). It is interesting to note that SAD standard treatment is 10,000 lux for 30 minutes at 12 inches from the light in the morning. As such, I was wondering where would be the healthiest part of the sky to look with the lowest amount of risk to damaging my eyes. I had damaged my eyes during researching the book "Solar Reflections for Architects, Engineers, and Human Health" and they took several months to recover. I did not want to have a similar experience!

So I looked at the anatomy of the skull. The eyes are recessed to prevent them from seeing the majority of the sky. So this indicated that the sky near to the horizon was the place to look. But what about high ultraviolet light (UV)? The least amount of UV is found looking away from the Sun. And what about the time of day to do this? I knew that I was dealing with an afternoon fatigue problem, so this indicated lunch time was the time to do this. So I decided to sit in a shady chair facing the pole (north in the northern hemisphere; south in the southern hemisphere) at noon every day, staring at the sky near to the polar horizon for half an hour and to see what happened. The first week was marked by severe insomnia, headaches and soft stools. By the second week these were subsiding and being replaced by afternoon energy! The third week I had excellent sleep patterns and good daytime energy levels. I was right, the sky near to the horizon could be used to offset radio frequency induced fatigue! I call this:

Horizon Polar Sky Fatigue Therapy

As the weeks progressed with the Horizon Polar Sky Fatigue Therapy I saw:

- Headaches.

- Occasions of afternoon fatigue.

- Pains in my lower right rib cage that subsided after a few weeks.

- Light induced impotence. I only saw one occurrence of this and it was during the time that extensive changes were occurring in my body from the light exposures.

These all cleared up several weeks later and I assume that they were in response to the many changes that were occurring in the human mind and body as it adapted to the blue sky irradiation of the blood and water systems. My sleep patterns continued to be excellent.

Regarding light induced impotence I can tell you that I have seen it before, I just did not know what was causing it. Typically after a long drive in the car where you spend most of the day looking at the horizon, when your normal routine is to be indoors. The significant shift in daylight radiation exposure to the eyes appears to cause it.

I came to the conclusion that blue light sensitivity that is extensively documented in medical literature is actually blue light deficiency. I could spend all day looking at the horizon blue sky and not see any insomnia. It was quite the opposite, I slept great!

In September 2014, I installed the radio frequency grounding system onto my electrical fuse board. I did it in weekly stages so that I could observe the biological reactions in the human:

- Week 1 – Installation of radio frequency ¾ inch copper plumbing grounding pipe. A 10 foot length of pipe was installed as the radio frequency ground from the fuse board and connected to the ground rod. The pipe was insulated by running it through flexible plastic plumbing drain tubing and the last couple of feet was exposed where it connected onto the ground rod. The end of the pipe was brought up to the surface to allow any remaining radio frequencies that wanted to leave the pipe for the surface of the earth. This was due to the "Skin Effect" of radio frequencies only liking to travel on the surface of things. A pipe bender was used to put smooth curves into the pipe, however, the one that I was sold was unsuitable for bending copper pipe and put kinks into the pipe. Highly stranded copper wire (cut up car battery booster cables) and two electrical pipe clamps were used to connect the copper pipe to the electrical fuse board ground terminals. An electrical direct burial pipe clamp was used to connect the copper pipe to the electrical ground cable near to the ground rod. I had some minor headaches after the installation of this for a few days. Due to the kinks in the pipe, I opted to install a second copper pipe radio frequency ground.

- Week 2 — Installation of additional radio frequency ¾ inch copper plumbing pipe. A 10 foot length of pipe was installed as the second radio frequency ground from the fuse board and connected to the ground rod. The pipe was insulated by running it through plastic tubing and the last couple of feet was exposed where it connected onto the ground rod. The end of the pipe was brought up to the surface about a foot away from the first pipe to allow any remaining radio frequencies that wanted to leave the pipe for the surface of the earth. It is preferable with multiple radio frequency grounding pipes to have them all different lengths, as each will likely be tuned to a different set of frequencies, similar to the pipes on an organ. 45 degree soldered angles were used to put smooth changes of direction into the pipe. I had some minor headaches after the installation of this for a few days.

- Week 3 – Installation of electrical grounding electrode system water irrigation. Grounding electrode systems work much better when they are in wet soil. As such, the grounding electrode system soil was soaked with water and irrigation drippers were installed to keep the area damp. The ground rods were automatically watered daily. I had some major headaches after the installation of this for a few days that required dosing with aspirin. My partner was also reporting general sickness that included a sore back and a sore throat, and a few days later I saw minor throat problems that seemed to interfere with my speaking.

- Week 4 – Watering with saltwater brine. Salt is cheap and is easily obtained in the hardware store as water softener salt. The salt was placed into a large bucket of water and it was left for several days to turn into saltwater brine. 5 gallons of saltwater brine was then slowly poured onto each of the ground rods. Gravity would take the saltwater brine to the full length of the ground rods. This greatly improves the conductivity of the grounding system. It may kill the plants or make them sickly in the areas that the saltwater brine goes into. Plants that are suitable for beach locations are more suited to high salt content soils and you should consider replacing your current plants in the area for these. Rain will wash away the saltwater brine and saltwater brine should be poured onto the ground rods to maintain good conductivity of the electrical grounding system after heavy rain. Take care with doing this, as you can be electrocuted by stray voltage coming in contact with the saltwater brine on your body! I had intestinal pains and loose stools during the following week.

- Week 5 – Installation of capacitive fuse board filter. Now that I had good radio frequency grounding, it was time to revisit capacitive filters. I installed 47.5 microfarad "Motor Run" capacitors between L1 to Nuetral, L2 to Neutral, and L1 to L2. These were Dayton part number 2GU39. It is a dual capacitor of 40 microfarad and 7.5 microfarad. The dual capacitors were wired in parallel to give the 47.5 microfarad rating.

Dual "Motor Run" capacitors are preferable for filtering purposes, as they will filter a wider range of frequencies than the standard "Motor Run" capacitors. The total capacitance was 142.5 microfarad. No health problems were observed. The electrical system was tested over 24 hours with a microsurge meter and was peaking over 90 GS units. It is recommended to keep the GS units below 50 which it was for most of the time.

- Week 6 - I installed 6 capacitors onto the fuse board to make a total of 285 microfarad of filtering capacitors. I also installed a whole home surge suppressor (Leviton 51110-1 120/240 Volt Panel Protector) at the fuse board. Testing showed that the surge suppressor had no effect on the GS readings of the microsurge meter. My partner reported congestion with headaches and sinus issues, and I showed lip problems and headaches. This cleared up after a few days. The electrical system was tested over 24 hours with a microsurge meter and was peaking to approximately 33 GS units.

- Week 7 – I installed 9 capacitors onto the fuse board to make a total of 427.5 microfarad of filtering capacitors. I had headaches, runny nose, sore lips, my speech was affected and my mother who was visiting also reported headaches. My 13 month old daughter's behavior was different and she was irritable, presumably because she had a headache. The electrical system was tested over 24 hours with a microsurge meter and was peaking to approximately 33 GS units, which was comparable to the previous week. There appears to be a limit where adding more capacitance is a health issue and this was exceeded above 142.5 microfarad. Too much capacitance seems to be a waste of money as it does not filter much better and this was reached at 285 microfarad on my electrical system.

- Week 8 – I reviewed my testing information and noted that the only capacitance that did not produce adverse health problems was 142.5 microfarad, so I went back to that and the surge protector. The headaches cleared up two days later.

- Weeks 9 to 12 – I did not see any adverse health affects.

- Week 13 to 15 – I developed daily headaches and a couple of weeks later I started to get tingling nerves in my face. As they were becoming more severe with time and that I had already established that large capacitors may cause headaches, I removed the 142.5 microfarad capacitive filter and this did not clear up the headaches and nerve problems. I stopped this testing in order to troubleshoot this health issue and it was unclear if the large microfarad capacitance had an effect in it or not.

There are no doubts that these changes to the home electrical system had postive effects on my health. After this testing the electrical fuse board was configured as follows:

- **Small fuse board capacitive filter that is detailed in the book "Electrical Forensics".**

- **Surge suppressor (Leviton 51110-1 120/240 Volt Panel Protector).**

- **Radio frequency electrical grounding copper pipes.**

- **Two 8 foot long electrical ground rods in wet soil.**

It is interesting to note that I have never been asked to do grounding electrode system maintenance by any employer throughout my career. I have never witnessed any company do grounding electrode system maintenance. Grounding systems are arguably the most important aspect of electrical engineering and it is poorly taught. Most electrical engineers in the USA think that pounding two ground rods into the earth and connecting them to the home fuse board with a #4 solid drawn copper cable is all that is required for an electrical grounding system. Such poor thinking may induce easily preventable sickness into your family.

Most electrical engineers do not own ground electrode testers and never test the electrical impedance of the electrical grounding systems that they are responsible for. This is despite it being well known by them that ground electrode systems must have a ground impedance of less than 25 ohms! Of the grounding systems that do get tested, it generally occurs when they are new. My National Electric Code (NEC) compliant home electrical ground rods (2 x 8 feet) were tested by the electrical utility company when they were new and they were about 14 ohms. A few years later they were about 140 ohms as they had aged, corroded, and dried out. A 140 ohm electrical grounding system is largely useless. I also found that the home foundation electrical grounding system (commonly called an Ufer) was largely useless, and this was due to the concrete being dry. The home foundation electrical ground tests well when the foundation is new and contains a lot of moisture, but degrades as the home foundation goes through long term corrosion and drying over several years. The National Electric Code (NEC) requires no testing of electrical ground rods, as long as there are two of them installed. This seems to be a very flawed policy, particularly in the desert southwest USA, a notoriously difficult area to achieve 25 ohm grounding systems.

Some people make the mistake of trying to achieve 1 ohm grounding systems. They put in lots of ground rods to get to this value. Do not try and do this on your home, as it electrifies the ground with stray voltage/currents/frequencies and may make you sick. The sweet spot with electrical grounding electrode systems appears to be below 25 ohms through to 1 ohm, this fact is well known to the electrical industry. The preference with home grounding is below 25 ohms, but not too far below. The very low 1 ohm grounding electrode systems are used for commercial purposes, such as industrial radio transmitters, electrical utility switch yards, substations, and lightning protection systems and you should avoid living near these due to the stray voltage/current/frequency troubles that they are known to cause.

If your electrical grounding system has not been designed for radio frequencies, then you should be concerned! Most home electrical ground rods use a #4 solid drawn copper cable to connect to the fuse board. A #4 solid drawn copper cable is terrible for carrying radio frequencies down to the ground rods. It is my opinion that home electrical grounding systems should use hollow copper pipes to connect the fuse board to wet ground rods to give an excellent radio frequency ground for mitigating dirty electricity effects.

During this grounding electrode research, I realized one of the reasons why I was getting occasional fatigue. I had known for years that some days I would see afternoon fatigue and other days I would be fine. I realized that it was the rain that would cause the fatigue to disappear. What happens in Tucson is that the dry earth changes to saturated earth and this makes all of the grounding electrode systems in the area to work as designed, each electrode system dropping below the required 25 ohm or lower standard. As the earth dries out, it slowly returns to the much higher impedance that does not meet the electric code standard. This brings with it the dirty electrical grounding that makes people sick! Low humidity and high temperatures equates to dirty electrical grounding systems in Tucson. The wireless radiation exposures to the electrical cables just adds to the dirty electrical grounding effects. It is the reason why you need the radio frequency grounding system on irrigation for good health.

To counteract the headaches and facial nerve pains that developed during this research, I again did the rouleaux flushing technique in November 2014. I did it differently this time to see if the side effects would be different also. I went straight onto the 650mg aspirin dosing (two tablets) every four hours and I did this for seven days. Some sleepiness showed up in the first few days and after seven days, the side effects showed up of not feeling well, headaches and strange dreams, so I reduced the dose down to nothing over two more days. I had extensive headaches during the following several weeks that required extra dosing of aspirin. The side effects were different compared to the first rouleaux flush

that I did and it would appear that my body had changed between the two times that I had used this health technique. This was consistent with no longer observing the extensive Electromagnetic Hypersensitivity symptoms after I did it the first time.

The definition between blood micro-clots and blood clots had emerged by this time:

- Blood Micro-clot: A blood micro-clot does not cause any apparent problems until the blood thickens. Once the blood has thickened, the effects of the micro-clots emerge and are apparent to the person. An example of this would be a person who sits near to a Wi-Fi router and starts to show adverse health symptoms that are cleared by moving away from the Wi-Fi router. The treatment is to move into a natural environment and to rouleaux flush.

- Blood Clot: A blood clot that causes problems to be observed continually until the clot is removed. An example of this would be a headache that will not clear up on its own. The treatment is to move into a natural environment and to rouleaux flush.

The detrimental blood clotting effects that showed up during this research have shed some light on how past extinctions, particularly the dinosaurs, may have occurred. It is clear that if the Earth's electromagnetic environment is significantly changed from natural levels, then the mammals may develop thickened blood. Thickened blood leads to micro-clots forming and micro-clots lead to blood clots. Lots of blood clots will lead to disease and possibly death. It is quite possible that a large shift in electromagnetic energy levels would wipe out entire species in a very short space of time. A large asteroid collision with the Earth would be one such event that could cause a sufficiently large shift and create "Extinction Energy". Another type of event is the rapid deployment of energy and radio frequency technology worldwide that results in a globally unnatural human electromagnetic environment. Unfortunately, we are currently in this event.

I was further able to improve my health by eating a strawberry jam sandwich for lunch. The sugar that this adds to the body generates afternoon energy. It appears that part of what I was experiencing was called "Reactive Hypoglycemia" (Low blood sugar in people who do not have diabetes). One can only wonder if radio frequency exposure and dirty electricity causes this condition?

By November 2014, it had become apparent that something had significantly changed within the home. I had been growing Dieffenbachia plants within the home since 2011 and my controls always deformed after six months of being in the home. My 2014 experiments that had started in March, April and May were not showing deformity. Rather, I was growing the best Dieffenbachia's that I have ever seen! This timing was inline with a radio frequency transmitter system being removed from the west antenna tower approximately 2,300 feet away and the heavy pruning of the largest tree on my property down from 30 feet to just 6 feet tall.

The long term effects of standing all day had started to show up with a sore heel on my right foot. It was only sore when I walked on it for the first ten minutes of every day. My doctor advised me to sit more during the day, which helped. The problem was reduced by wearing athletic shoes with good arch support during my daytime standing. I had been previously wearing slippers that had no support in them. To prevent problems from standing all day, I also make sure that I take regular walking and sitting breaks during the day.

I had my vitamin D tested and it was 29, the normal range starts at 30. So I had to further increase my outdoor time. I was already spending at least an hour outdoors daily, so I increased it by another half an hour by sunbathing. I spent 15 minutes on my front and 15 minutes on my back. I did this at a time of day that was warm so that I sweated and the Sun was weak enough that I did not need to use sunscreen. I found that this eventually brought on hot and sore skin and this leads to me to conclude that my English genetics are simply not adapted to

Arizona direct sunlight exposure, the higher radiation levels in the sunlight are far too harsh for my fair skin. So I increased my outdoor shade time by half an hour instead.

I had known for a long time that the days that I spent outdoors were great, but the days spent indoors were not so good. This indicated that something was wrong inside of the home. I eventually noticed that the whole home was very, very quiet. The home has approximately 2 feet of insulation in the attic, 5 inches of insulation in the walls and double glazed windows which make the home silent. As such, I wanted noise inside of the home. I knew that extensive plant research had been done by playing different types of music to them. The conclusion was that classical music gave the best growth patterns. So I started to play classical music daily from the point where I would get up until bedtime. I placed the speakers in the center of the home and played the music loud enough that I could hear it throughout the home. This had the effect of improving my mental clarity and energy levels.

I decided to test the home for sound levels using a sound meter. The meter reads decibels (dB) and has an A scale that matches the sensitivity of the human ear in normal environments and a C scale that matches the sensitivity of the human ear in really loud areas, such as pop music concerts. The C scale is more sensitive than the human ear in normal environments. Why the two settings are not referred to as "normal" and "loud" is a mystery of the sound industry. This is what I found in the afternoon:

- Indoors, no music playing:
  - A = Less than 40 dB.
  - C = 40 dB to 60 dB pulsing.
- Indoors, classical music playing:
  - A = 45 dB average & 51 dB maximum.
  - C = 50 dB average & 65 dB maximum.
- Outdoors:

- A = 40 dB average & 47 dB maximum.

- C = 50 dB average & 63 dB maximum.

As you can see, the home was more comparable to outdoors with the classical music playing. I was not able to ascertain what was causing the pulsing on the C scale when no music was playing inside of the home.

I decided to investigate the effects of sound on the human mind and body further and I used the following products:

- Timex "nature sounds" clock radio.

- 3-Tier bronze stone contemporary tabletop fountain.

- LectroFan - fan sound and white noise machine.

I had wondered what would happen if I played sounds continuously, so I started sleeping with sounds. The first night I slept listening to the classical music radio station. I had a terrible nights sleep and this seemed to be due to the sound of the DJ chatting. It seems that the human is designed to wake up to the sound of voices. The second night I slept to the nature sound of ocean waves. Again, I slept terribly and this seemed to be due to the sound of birds on the soundtrack. Birds sleep during the night, so the unnatural nighttime sound of the birds seemed to be waking me up. The third night I slept to the sound of a flowing stream and got an excellent nights sleep. I continued to sleep to this sound for a week and had excellent sleep and wonderful daytime energy levels. I did notice:

- Some head pains and minor headaches towards the end of the first week of testing and I assumed that these were due to the changed environmental conditions.

- Some aches and pains from my upper abdomen.

- A high pitched, really loud screeching in my ears that would come and go.

- If I woke up in the night to urinate, then I sometimes could not get back to sleep.

- The second week of testing was marked by insomnia and interrupted sleep patterns. This cleared up in the third week.

I switched out the Timex "nature sounds" clock radio for the tabletop fountain. The fountain had a nice loud flow of water to it. It was so loud that I could not have it in the bedroom with me! So I moved it out next to the front door and this gave a nice low background sound of running water in the bedrooms. The advantage of this location was that it would fill the entire home with the sound of running water. I was listening to classical radio music during the daytime only and the fountain was on continuously. The afternoon fatigue had completely disappeared during this week of testing.

I switched out the table top fountain for the LectroFan. The LectroFan comes with ten fan sounds and ten white noise sounds. I decided to use the *"lowest pitch white noise"* setting for my testing, as this seemed to be the most pleasant of the sounds that the unit produced. I placed the unit near the front door and had it just loud enough so that I could hear it in the bedroom. I was listening to classical radio music during the daytime and the LectroFan was on continuously. I found that it was much more agreeable to fall asleep to and that I slept really well.

It had become apparent that strange mental patterns which I noticed occurring shortly after moving into my home in 2007 had subsided. This mental pattern was largely one of apathy, I did not seem to be motivated to do things that were important to me. This resulted in a very messy and disorganized home office. I could never get motivated to keep it organized and clean, even though it was important to me. This apathy cleared up and my office was finally tidied after many years of being a mess. I had never experienced such good mental clarity in this home!

After indoor sound testing was complete, I decided to keep the home filled with sounds. I now use the following:

- Daytime only: Classical radio music and the water fountain were used to create normal noise levels for the human (45-50 Decibels).

- Daytime & nighttime: LectroFan played continuously at background noise levels (40-45 Decibels).

After this testing, it had become clear that silence was hazardous to human health and extended periods in silent areas should be avoided. It appears that the inner ear and the human skin should always be in an area that is at least 40 to 50 decibels to enable them to be sufficiently vibrating from the pressure of the sound waves. The lack of these vibrations seems to bring on sickness. Silence appears to be one of nature's secret biological weapons against invasive species. Any species that devours its natural environment will eventually fall victim to the resulting silence and I call the toxicity of silence:

Extinction Silence

The health benefits of music have been observed and documented in both plants and humans. The book "The Secret Life of Plants: a Fascinating Account of the Physical, Emotional, and Spiritual Relations Between Plants and Man" documents how plants respond well to classical music. Indeed, during this sound testing I had noticed experimental Dieffenbachia plants that were extremely stressed and on the verge of death in my home mysteriously coming back to life! In some of the stressed plants, it appeared to revitalize the sickly pale light green leaves to the dark green chlorophyll filled leaves. I do wonder if vitamin D and other nutrients associated with light exposure in the human body are related to natural sounds as well as natural light. The documentary

"Alive Inside" details *"music's ability to combat memory loss and restore a deep sense of self"* in sick humans.

In December 2014 I suddenly became very irritable. One day I was fine, the next I was reacting to little things that would not normally bother me. It came on very quickly and after two days of this, I became suspicious that the radio frequencies had changed around my home, as irritability in radio wave fields is extensively documented. I took a walk around the outside of my property and found very high radio frequency (RF) levels to the north of my home that were not there the last time I tested the area. I was finding levels of over 700 millivolts per meter (mV/m), this exceeds the international environmental standard of 614 mV/m. So I increased my supplementation and moved away from this hot-zone of RF radiation. The irritability completely disappeared within a day.

Since the last rouleaux flush, I had been struggling with daily headaches. They did not appear to be radio frequency headaches, as they were distinctly different from what I saw during my Electromagnetic Hypersensitivity experience. I had been treating them with aspirin and Alka-Seltzer. However, they would not clear up. I eventually realized that it was a side effect of prolonged supplementation. My plants that had previously been deforming in the biologically toxic radio wave fields had stopped deforming and were now growing normally. This indicated that the atmospheric DC voltage had been restored at my home and that I no longer needed to supplement for DC body voltage. So I stopped the supplements and watched. This is what happened:

- Cold symptoms of sore throat, runny nose and sneezing showed up and appeared to be withdrawal symptoms that lasted over a week.

- Within two weeks the headaches were gone.

- Normal health patterns with no fatigue whatsoever appeared after the headaches cleared up.

My health by the end of December 2014 was relatively normal with some lasting memory effects, short term memory problems being the primary issue. These were the lasting injuries from the biologically toxic brain exposures that I received in 2009 from the weird electromagnetic energy fields at the high powered solar photovoltaic utility generation system. The buzzing ears continue and are a feature of everyone living in this home. I now live life with a recognition that I live in a very unnatural radiation environment. Some of the health techniques that I routinely use are comparable to what are in use on the International Space Station (ISS) to protect astronauts against the long term damaging effects of unnatural Space radiation exposures and Faraday cage effects.

It is interesting to note that in 2014 I consumed approximately 300 aspirin 325mg tablets and 150 Alka-Seltza tablets during the year to develop the research. My urine pH was 9, which meant that my body had alkalized. pH of 9 is commonly reported in people who live organic lifestyles and these people are known for their good health. Most of the modern population have a pH of 7.

At the age of 44 I had cleared up almost all of the health conditions that I had accumulated over the years. All that was left was the buzzing ears. My partner does not have Electromagnetic Hypersensitivity but does have the buzzing ears. I have to conclude that I went into remission from Electromagnetic Hypersensitivity in 2014.

It had become clear that my toddler was remarkably healthy, as compared to her counterparts. She had rarely been sick during fifteen months and her growth for head circumference and length was in the 50th percentile. Interestingly, she was unusually light and was in the 17th percentile for weight. She routinely slept from 20:00 through to 10:00 and would sleep from 14:00 to 17:00. It was rare for her to wake up in the middle of the night. She did not appear to be skinny, just very happy and healthy. She had been getting comparable environmental exposures to me, as I was her full time parent. Her counterparts had multiple occurrences of sickness and were heavier in their first year. It appeared that the daily outdoor light exposures were a significant factor in this remarkably good health. Dr. John Nash Ott was right, correct outdoor light exposures result in really good health!

Again Jesus spoke to them, saying, "I am the light of the world. Whoever follows me will not walk in darkness, but will have the light of life."

John 8:12

Biological Problems in Tucson

The bulk of the research in this book was performed in Tucson, Arizona, USA. What surprised me was the level of biological toxicity that this town presents to the unsuspecting human. My impression from dealing with the local utilities and government regulators is that my home is simply typical of the average American home! This also matches my assessment of homes that I have performed measurements in around the Tucson area. The problems at my home appear to be quite mild when compared to others that I have visited in the southwest. I find this very concerning. The problems of Tucson are:

- Stray voltage/currents/frequencies on tiled flooring, toilets, sinks, baths and showers from the electrical utility grounding system and utility services in the street. Some gardens and trees are radiating biologically harmful electromagnetic energy from the electrified ground that they are planted into. The electrical utility and Arizona Corporation Commission refuses to fix these known problems, even though they deform garden plants and houseplants. They know human sickness occurs with prolonged exposure to it.

- Utility high voltage power lines and poles in the area are emitting a wide range of electromagnetic radiation. Long term exposure to these emissions may make you sick. The utility electrical distribution system is poorly maintained.

- The State of Arizona has passed laws that override home owners association rules. Unfortunately, people in home owners associations throughout Arizona are inadvertently finding out that some of their home owners association rules and regulations are largely useless at protecting their health and safety rights.

- Neighbor's wireless radiation emissions including their transmitting utility meters. The gas utility, Arizona

Corporation Commission and the Federal Communications Commission are known to refuse to remove biologically toxic radio frequency transmitting utility meters from the vicinity of homes of people who are experiencing adverse health symptoms, even though they may have a doctors letter stating that they should not be exposed to these radiation emissions. The utilities and government are completely okay with their electronic harassment of vulnerable individuals.

- People who have been made sick by radio frequency transmitting utility meters are expected to be charged an "Opt Out Fee" in the near future, even though they never opted in. That is to say, a bio-hazard that was created by the utility companies that damaged some of their customers health will be removed if the sick customer pays what amounts to a "Healthy Home Extortion Fee". The radio frequency transmitting utility meters that will be removed are the ones at their property, their neighbors meters will remain in service and continue to pollute the property with known biologically harmful radio frequency transmissions. If the person has gas, water and electricity, then these fees may approach $100 extra on their monthly utility bills for a person who has been made sick by the utility companies, may have lost their job, is accumulating expensive medical fees and may die prematurely from radiation induced diseases.

- The State of Arizona uses incorrect test equipment in their studies of the radiated power levels of radio frequency transmitting utility meters. They use a radio frequency meter that has no ability to accurately record the true peak values of microsecond and millisecond duration pulsed radio frequency radiation. They do not seem to use a radio frequency meter that has been certified by a Nationally Recognized Testing Laboratory (NRTL). This certification of test equipment is generally required for legal work regarding public health and safety. Unfortunately, most electromagnetic radiation researchers own a higher specification of radio frequency power level meter than what the State of Arizona uses for determining public health and safety standards!

• The State of Arizona does not appear to have studied the full range of radio frequency transmitting utility system devices. Some of the components that seem to have been conveniently omitted are radio frequency transmitting car mounted meter readers, radio frequency solar photovoltaic meters, radio frequency network node meters and radio frequency network repeaters commonly mounted on streetlights and power poles outside of homes. The items that I identified as being really biologically toxic were the Itron 100G gas meter and a close exposure to the car mounted radio frequency transmitting meter reader was by far the most biologically toxic device to the human.

• There is no disclosure of the known adverse health effects that radio frequency transmitting utility meters are known to have on human health. While documented in the State of Arizona public records, this information is not disclosed by the various utilities installing the radio frequency transmitting utility meters on people's homes and workplaces. This leaves vulnerable individuals unaware that their deteriorating health is related to the radio frequency transmitting utility meters and they typically get a misdiagnosis from the medical profession with expensive prescription medications.

• The electrical utilities are known to install radio frequency transmitting utility meters without switching the power to the home off. Such activity is a health and safety hazard and may damage the fuse board electrical connections, may eventually cause meter electrical connection arcing, arcing radio frequency emissions, overheating of the meter and eventually fire. Fires regarding these radio frequency transmitting electrical meters are extensively documented.

- The radio frequency radiation environment of Tucson, Arizona, is heavily overloaded by many forms of wireless communication systems. The city appears to have radio frequency levels that averages around 1,000 mV/m and peaks to over 2,000 mV/m at homes and businesses that I have measured. The Tenmars TM-196 RF meter manual states *"We recommend a maximum level of 614 mV/m for prolonged exposure"*.

- Irresponsible siting of radio frequency infrastructure. You will find cell phone towers located in the middle of dense residential neighborhoods and cell phone transmitters on the corners of tall residential apartment buildings and tall hotels. You should expect higher rates of sickness in people who live close to these areas. The City of Tucson does not even know what the RF power levels are in these areas, despite permitting the RF infrastructure!

- I have attended a number of cell phone tower planning hearings and I can confirm that the City of Tucson does not allow residents to submit evidence regarding the known biological toxicity of cell phone towers! They refuse to put it into the public records, even from people who have been made sick by them. They know that they are making people sick and they are keeping this fact out of the City of Tucson public records. Cell phone towers are generally regarded as increasing the health and safety risks to people who live within a quarter of a mile of them and the risks typically increase the closer a person lives to the tower.

- The City of Tucson is permitting radio frequency transmitters on Tucson Water properties. This is concerning, as we know that irradiating water with radio frequencies changes the biological structure of it.

- Sonic boom infra-sound waves passing through the area. The military bombing range is not moving any time soon.

- RADAR, chemical trails, sonic roars, sonic pulsations, communications emissions from military helicopters and airplanes that are routinely flying low over Tucson and the surrounding areas. These are not leaving Tucson any time soon. Living in Tucson is like living in a country at war, due to the very large military airbase and nearby bombing range.

- Excessive lightning strikes. The east side of Tucson appears to be the worst for high rates of lightning strikes and I recommend that people should avoid living on that side of the town. Lightning strikes generate electromagnetic radiation emissions of many types that may result in biological harm to vulnerable individuals.

- Many homes have energy saving tinted windows. The long term health problems from exposure to filtered light from such windows is poorly documented and will depend on the tint used.

- Many homes are heavily insulated and are silent inside. We know that long term exposure to silence is harmful to human health.

I have successfully adapted to the list of biologically toxic environmental conditions above, however, I do plan on moving away from Tucson in the long term to protect my family's health. Protecting my family's health is something that the State of Arizona has opted not to do.

"Adapt or perish, now as ever, is nature's inexorable imperative."

H. G. Wells

Summary

There are no doubts that we are all alive during a very toxic era of humanity. This toxic era is inducing a wide range of preventable illness and disease into many people. The new wave of Electromagnetic Hypersensitivity appearing in the modern world populations is a very concerning development that is a product of this toxic era.

Modern society has turned into one of great deceit of the masses by massive corporations and their modern corporate governments that they sponsor. It is likely that your family's medical conditions are easily preventable, but it is far more profitable to have you in a sick or diseased state. Irradiation of the human by the many forms of electromagnetic radiation results in your family purchasing medical care, visiting highly paid doctors, taking expensive drugs, and a likely decline into disease. You may actually live a very long life in a poorly functioning state, as radiation exposures are known to extend the human life span by stressing the cellular system.

We have to thank the USA corporate government for their known biologically toxic Smart/AMR/AMI radio frequency transmitting utility meter program and the USA utilities that have installed it. They prompted a wide range of people who became sick from exposure to these biologically toxic emissions to explore the world of electromagnetic radiation induced sickness. Like many people who became sick, I found that researching man-made radiation immersed me into a corporate world of lie, confuse and deny. At the point where lying, confusing and denying stopped working for them, they became silent. This is the last line of defense in the corporate world. I recommend the book "Doubt is Their Product: How Industry's Assault on Science Threatens Your Health" by David Michaels for more information on this delusional corporate world.

I would suggest that it is in your interest to practice prudent avoidance of man-made radiation sources, such as electricity, electronics, and wireless radiation. You may need to be supplementing for "Radiation Resistance". My radiation resistance supplementation routine is shown below (brand used is in brackets). It is a two part process. The charging process is used first until the body becomes fully charged with the supplements. The charging process should be stopped once supplementing overdosing is observed. The charging process is then replaced with the floating process.

Charging process:

Breakfast:

- Cup of coffee. (Organic natural coffee beans that are ground with a home grinder).

- One multivitamin capsule (Twinlab Daily Two Caps with Iron).

- One 250mg magnesium tablet (Country Life Chelated Magnesium).

- One 600mg kelp capsule (Natures Way Kelp).

- Electrolyte capsule (Saltstick Caps).

- One teaspoon of brewers yeast (Twinlab Genuine Brewers Yeast).

- One teaspoon of psyllium husk (Metamucil).

Lunch:

- One teaspoon of edible Bentonite Clay (Redmond Clay).

- Pot of hot organic tea. (Use various organic teas during the week).

- Organic strawberry jam sandwich.

Dinner:

- One multivitamin capsule (Twinlab Daily Two Caps with Iron).

- Cup of organic caffeine-free herbal tea (Use various organic teas during the week).

Supper:

- Electrolyte capsule (Succeed! S!Caps).

Daily:

- Spend the day standing outdoors in the shade or stand near to a shady ultraviolet transmitting window in a bright room all day long. Avoid sitting down.

- Walk in sunlight for half an hour (No sunglasses, no glasses, no contact lenses, no sunscreen. If the Sun is too strong, use clothing and hats to reduce the strength. It is preferable to do this walk in the shade of trees.)

- Horizon Polar Sky Fatigue Therapy at noon for half an hour.

- Exercise to convert fat to muscle mass.

- Walk barefoot in areas where the ground and atmosphere is not contaminated by man-made electromagnetic radiation. Do not do this if there is lightning in the area!

- Eat lots of organic fresh fruits and vegetables. Keep meat and fish to about 6% total of your dietary intake.

- Avoid areas of high levels of wireless radiation.

- Only use the electrical and electronic products that you absolutely need to.

- Avoid areas of pollution.

- When indoors, ensure you are in an area that has good ventilation to the outdoors.

- When indoors, ensure that you are in a natural sound filled environment.

- Wear a battery powered wristwatch with a resin strap and a second hand (Casio MW-600).

- Use rotational sleeping.

- Avoid spending time above 4,900 feet.

Weekly:

- Tablespoon of fish oil (Twinlab Norwegian Cod Liver Oil).

- Tablespoon of natural organic pure honey.

- Pint of stout (Home brewed is the best).

- 1,916mg Sodium bicarbonate, 325mg aspirin, anhydrous citric acid 1,000mg (One Alka-Seltza tablet).

Yearly:

- Consider hibernating for a few weeks or months in winter.

As needed:

- Rouleaux flushing.

The floating process is similar to above except that the daily supplementing techniques change to much lower levels.

Floating Process:

Monday, Wednesday & Friday:

Breakfast:

- Cup of coffee. (Organic natural coffee beans that are ground with a home grinder).
- One teaspoon of brewers yeast (Twinlab Genuine Brewers Yeast).
- Quarter of a teaspoon of Mediterranean sea salt (Trader Joe's Sea Salt).

Lunch:

- Pot of hot organic tea (Use various organic teas during the week).
- Organic strawberry jam sandwich.

Dinner:

- One multivitamin capsule (Twinlab Daily Two Caps with Iron).
- One 500 mG seaweed capsule (Seagate Seaweed).

Tuesday, Thursday & Saturday:

Breakfast:

- Cup of coffee. (Organic natural coffee beans that are ground with a home grinder).
- One teaspoon of psyllium husk (Metamucil).
- Quarter of a teaspoon of Mediterranean sea salt (Trader Joe's Sea Salt).

Lunch:

- Pot of hot organic tea (Use various organic teas during the week).

- Organic strawberry jam sandwich.

Dinner:

- One 250mg magnesium tablet (Country Life Chelated Magnesium).

- One 600mg kelp capsule (Natures Way Kelp).

Sunday:

Breakfast:

- Cup of coffee. (Organic natural coffee beans that are ground with a home grinder).

- Quarter of a teaspoon of Mediterranean sea salt (Trader Joe's Sea Salt).

Lunch:

- One Teaspoon of edible Bentonite Clay (Redmond Clay).

- Pot of hot organic tea (Use various organic teas during the week).

You may need to switch from the floating process to the charging process from time to time for short periods. After charging the human body, I would only revert from floating back to charging if I was seeing degrading health. After charging and floating the human body, you may be able to take a prolonged break from these processes if you are no longer experiencing Electromagnetic Hypersensitivity.

All drinking water should be boiled and stored in a water pitcher that has a teaspoon of edible clay in the bottom of it in order to mineralize that water.

People familiar with the charging of batteries will recognize these terms as those used in lead acid battery maintenance. It became clear during my research that the human body appears to be a rechargeable battery that is charged from the atmospheric DC voltage and by being barefoot in contact with the ground. The charging process can also be effected chemically by ingesting metals and electrolytes, as these are the ingredients of DC batteries.

This is what the charging and floating processes are doing:

- Standing all day: This keeps the body in tension, burns calories and changes the radio frequency characteristics of it.

- Metals (multivitamin & magnesium) and electrolytes (salts): This creates a DC voltage on the human body between the soles of the feet and the index finger of approximately 0.5 volt DC. It changes the electrical conductivity of the body.

- Clay: Offsets the demineralization effects of radio frequency exposure on the water systems of the human mind and body.

- Yeast, seaweed, fish oil, honey and stout: Provides the body with essential nutrients and micro-nutrients that have been lost through modern farming and food processing techniques.

- Tea & kelp: These appear to create radiation resistance in the body for reasons that are currently unknown. The kelp provides iodine to the thyroid to offset radiation damage to it.

- Psyllium husk: Provides fiber to the digestive tract to offset radio frequency effects on it.

- Sunlight exposures: There are extensive photosynthesis processes taking place when you expose the human eyes and skin to the Sun and the shade of trees. These are essential to good human health and vitamin D production.

- Horizon Polar Sky Fatigue Therapy: The eyes irradiate the blood and water systems of the human body. This appears to offset the fatigue aspect of radio frequency exposure.

- Converting fat to muscle mass: This changes the electrical characteristics of the body to increased radio frequency tolerance.

- Eating fresh and organic: This food has the highest nutritional content and will nourish the mind and body.

- Walking barefoot: Increases the natural DC charging of the human battery from the atmosphere. It creates a DC pulse on the human body with every step. Both appear to improve radiation resistance.

- Wearing a battery powered analogue watch: Simulates walking barefoot by creating a DC pulse on the human body with each movement of the second hand.

- Rotational sleeping: There are electromagnetic radiation biological hotspots within homes. Rotational sleeping ensures that your brain is not subjected to these hotspots continually during sleep.

- Rouleaux flushing: This clears out blood clots and micro-clots from the brain that have been formed by radio frequency exposure.

- Jam Sandwich: Taken at solar noon creates a surge in blood sugars and this helps prevent the afternoon fatigue slump occurring.

- Indoor natural sounds: The classical music stimulates the ears and brain. White noise and flowing water bring the outdoors inside. The sound pressure waves interact with the mind and body to create an environment comparable to outdoors which leads to good health.

I was able to stop the charging and floating processes after the atmospheric DC voltage reappeared at my home in 2014. The atmospheric DC charging of the human body was restored and I went into normal health without the need for supplementation. I can only wonder what would have happened to my long term health had I not discovered that the atmospheric DC voltage had gone missing and used the human body DC battery charging techniques to replace it.

Radiation resistance techniques will likely offset some of the illness that modern society is inducing into your family. You should consult with a licensed and practicing doctor and adjust the techniques to work for your particular health situation.

During the research, it emerged that there are very distinct areas of the human that are being affected by radio frequency exposure:

- Brain.
- Head & Neck:

  ○ Hearing is the most affected with buzzing ears being the common report. Some people report hearing things.

  ○ Eyes are known for their sensitivity to radio frequencies and may become irritated.

  ○ Smell can be significantly affected. You may think you are smelling things that are not present.

  ○ Voice can be affected, making it difficult to talk.

  ○ Skin on the head may get painful with random pins and needles sensations with hot skin that feels like sunburn.

- Heart.
- Digestive tract.
- Skin.

Stray voltage/currents/frequencies on the flooring and drains also appeared to have these effects:

- Irritability.
- Disturbed sleep patterns.
- Insomnia.
- Heart arrhythmia.
- Cracked skin on the feet.
- Occasional loss of toe nails.
- Sore feet.
- Sore knees.
- Urethra problems.

Sleeping near to electrified trees appeared to have these effects:

- Strange dreams.
- Chronic Fatigue.

You will not find me sleeping in Faraday cages, living in foil lined rooms or wondering around in electromagnetically shielded clothing. I have concerns about the long term health effects of these techniques and I recommend people to avoid using them until more is known on the subject. There is a time and place for electromagnetic shielding and I regard it as a last resort due to the long term biological problems that I have observed with it over the years in plant growth experiments. Plants show long term growth defects near it. I have never heard of

an electromagnetically hypersensitive person recovering from the condition using shielding and Faraday cages, they just seem to become social lepers due to their increasing reactivity to the city environment and addicts to their shielded environment. There were three people in my home and I was the only one showing Electromagnetic Hypersensitivity and reactivity to the radio frequency transmitting utility meters. For these reasons I did not shield my home and took the route of adapting my body to the toxic electromagnetic environment.

Most large telescope facilities are essentially Faraday cages and I am seeing extensive biological damage occurring in plants that are grown inside of Faraday cages and they eventually die. The world's largest telescope facility is now being constructed at high altitude, called the Thirty Meter Telescope (TMT). TMT needs to understand the long term implications of these effects on its workers, it is the law. It is interesting to note that the W. M. Keck Observatory where I worked does not have a medical person in the summit team to track and document health effects in their high altitude staff. As far as I am aware, no one has been studying the long term health effects of high altitude exposure on workers from the W. M. Keck Observatory, the partner to the TMT, and I find this very concerning as there are clearly long term health problems associated with working there.

Remote National Parks offer the ability to assess if your health symptoms are being caused by electrical exposures, transmitter systems and window glazing in your environment. Most transmitter systems are banned from National Parks and that includes cell phone towers. So take a camping trip and engage in outdoor activities for a few weeks and see if your health improves there. Be careful though, as you may initially go into withdrawal! The withdrawal will be similar to cold and flu symptoms and should clear up after a week or so.

In 2009 the doctors could not diagnose what was wrong with me, they were telling me that I was getting old and it was a normal aspect of aging. I now know that they were misleading me, as what I had was not a normal aspect of aging. My health was at its worst in 2009 and I could only work due to taking prescription drugs. Without the drugs I would have been constantly laying in bed day and night and unable to work. I no longer need any prescription drugs of any kind and I have excellent sleep patterns. My health is now recovered. There is only one reason why I am relatively healthy today and that is because I detoxified from the radiation exposures after discovering that I had radiation sickness.

The high radio frequency radiation levels matches the abnormal growth patterns that I have observed in the Dieffenbachia (Dumb Cane) plants. For years I could only get them to show improved growth patterns that are similar to the original growth by connecting them to 1.5 volt batteries, grounding the pot to the closest tiled floor to my back garden, putting battery powered resin strap wristwatches in the roots, watering with tea, and giving them human vitamin and mineral supplements. Without this type of intervention, they were showing excessive deformity. In 2014 the electromagnetic environment of the home clearly changed and I can now grow the Dieffenbachia in my home without any intervention. This matched the timing of my largest tree being heavily pruned and a transmitter going missing from the west antenna tower. Despite making inquiries, no one will inform me what that transmitter was and what the remaining transmitters are, these are secrets of the USA government, the Federal Communications Commission (FCC) and the wireless industry.

Based on what I have seen with these Dieffenbachia plants, I have to conclude that modern cities and suburban areas have a level of biological toxicity associated with them. This toxicity is increasing with each year of the wireless revolution. This matches what we are seeing in the children. Autism is an accelerating disease in the children and there are no doubts today that electromagnetic interference exposures are driving it. The children are like the coalminers canary in the cage, when they are not developing properly, you know you have got some really serious human environmental problems!

It is interesting to note that the Electromagnetic Hypersensitivity health techniques developed in this book compare well with those reported by the atomic bomb survivors of Japan. I came to the conclusion that there really is not much biological difference between exposure to low levels of radioactive ionizing radiation and the non-ionizing radiation that electrical, electronics and wireless products produce, which is commonly called *"Electromagnetic Interference (EMI)"*.

Domestic terrorism is alive and well in the USA and it is masquerading as "Progress". While the USA government and the corporate media will advise you that you are involved in a "War on Terror", they are lying, confusing and denying that they are willfully toxifying society at the expense of your health. Unfortunately, you are far more likely to be harmed or die prematurely as a direct result of modern society than you are from any form of terrorism.

So, as you can see, I have had quite a journey through the realms of human health issues. My conclusion is that the majority of ailments that humans suffer from are caused by incorrect environmental exposures. Both sunlight and electrical systems are sources of radiation exposures and you need to be aware of your exposure to these.

You should spend time characterizing your body and establish the correct daily level of outdoor sunlight exposure for it. You should also characterize your electrical environment and reduce your exposures as much as possible to electrical systems and products. You should only have the exposures that are absolutely necessary in order to do what you need to do. The more exposures you have to electricity then the more likely it is to impact your health. These health effects appear in most people as general poor health and compromised mental functioning.

Regarding children, you should avoid purchasing electrical, electronic and wireless toys for them. It is preferable to also turn off the electrical circuit in their bedroom. Developing children should not be sleeping in rooms that have electricity in them. Do not purchase a television or laptop computer for their rooms, as the

electromagnetic fields are too large for their developing cells to cope with in the long term. With developing children you should be keeping their environment as natural as possible.

It is preferable to arrange your rooms and use common sense so that you are not exposed to easily avoidable electromagnetic fields. Some simple steps are:

- Do not walk barefoot on conductive flooring that has stray voltage on it.

- Do not urinate into toilets that have stray voltage on the water.

- Keep chairs away from walls.

- Avoid putting chairs within 10 feet of a television in all directions.

- Be aware of what products are on the other side of the walls.

- Do not put chairs near to large appliances like cookers, microwave ovens, refrigerators, washers and dryers.

- Stay away from electrical fuse boards and utility meters.

- Be aware of what is under the floor on upper story's and avoid the electromagnetic hotspots that may appear in the floor.

- Use wooden furniture.

- Sleep on a natural foam mattress on a low wooden bed frame far away from the electrical fuse board and utility transmitting meters. It is preferable for the bed to be in the center of the room to keep it away from the electrical cables in the wall.

- Your bedroom should be free of electricity and electrical, electronic and wireless products.

- Do not use radioactive ionizing smoke detectors, have photoelectric ones instead.

- Do not use wireless products.

- Use only the electrical and electronic products that you need. Unplug them when not in use.

- Use full spectrum filament light bulbs for daytime lighting.

- Use standard filament light bulbs for nighttime lighting.

- Remove trees and climbing vines that are near to bedrooms that may be emitting harmful electromagnetic interference due to electrification from wireless radiation and stray voltage/currents/frequencies in the ground.

- Cut down your garden to about 1 foot tall if it is electrified with wireless radiation or stray voltage/currents/frequencies to reduce the biologically harmful electromagnetic interference emissions.

- Avoid spending time near to refrigerators, fans and air conditioning units, as their "Motor Run" capacitors and associated wiring may be emitting biologically harmful radio frequencies.

- Be aware of the transmitters in your local neighborhood.

- Pay attention to the locations of transformers, streetlights and power poles near your home.

I advise people not to live in "Energy Star" homes and homes that have double glazing, tinted windows, electronic light bulbs and high levels of insulation. These appear to have long term toxicity implications to the human. If you do live in such a home I advise:

- Removal of the tint from the windows.

- Change shady windows to ultraviolet transmitting acrylic single pane windows.

- Change all electronic light bulbs to filament.

- Install air vents on north, east, west and south walls, and all bedrooms to allow the sounds and fresh air from outdoors to come into the home.

- Introduce sounds throughout the home in the form of daytime classical music and running water at normal levels in the daytime living areas and at a low background level in the bedrooms. Background white noise should be on continuously in the home.

- Whenever possible, open the windows to bring the outdoors inside.

- Have Dieffenbachia plants throughout the home to humidify the home. These will shows stress and deformity if the environment is toxic and will alert you to problems within the home.

Good health for most people is easy to achieve and it just takes some simple adjustments in lifestyle. The adjustments are far easier than expensive visits to the doctor and mentally challenged children.

I would like to sum up this book with a very prophetic statement made by Nikola Tesla:

"You may live to see man-made horrors beyond your comprehension."

Nikola Tesla

References

- Alive Inside: http://www.aliveinside.us/
- Bell Hooks.
- Bible.
- Bill Gates.
- Camilla Rees, MBA.
- Centers for Disease Control and Prevention: http://www.cdc.gov/
- Columbia University: http://www.columbia.edu/
- Dartmouth College: http://dartmouth.edu/
- Devra Davis.
- Dr. John Nash Ott.
- Dr. Magda Havas.
- Dr. William Rea.
- Earl Wilson.
- Elizabeth Kelley MA.
- Eric Schmidt.
- Erma Bombeck.
- Galileo Galilei.
- Greenwave: http://www.greenwavefilters.com/
- H. G. Wells.
- Henry Ward Beecher.
- Isaac Newton Group of Telescopes: http://www.ing.iac.es/

- Joyce Carol Oates.

- Ken Goldberg.

- Les Brown.

- Martin Pall.

- MDM Observatory: http://mdm.kpno.noao.edu/

- NASA: http://www.nasa.gov/

- Nikola Tesla.

- Royal Liverpool University Hospital:
  http://www.rlbuht.nhs.uk/OurHospitals/Pages/Royal
  %20Liverpool%20University%20Hospital.aspx

- Science and Technology Facilities Council:
  http://www.stfc.ac.uk/Home.aspx

- Stetzer Electric: http://www.stetzerelectric.com/

- The Earthing Institute:
  http://www.earthinginstitute.net/

- The Secret Life of Plants by Peter Thomkins &
  Christopher Bird.

- Thirty Meter Telescope (TMT): http://www.tmt.org/

- Tracing EMF's in Building Wiring and Grounding
  by Karl Riley.

- University of California:
  http://www.universityofcalifornia.edu/

- Wikipedia: http://www.wikipedia.org/

- W. M. Keck Observatory:
  http://www.keckobservatory.org/

- World Health Organization: http://www.who.int/en/

"None of us is as smart as all of us."
Eric Schmidt

Internet

Manufacturers of ultraviolet (UV) transmitting full spectrum acrylic window glazing sheets are:

Lucite International, Inc: LuciteLux UTRAN UVT:
http://www.lucitelux.com/product.aspx?productID=4

Spartech: Solacryl "Monkey-Shine" SUVT:
http://www.spartech.com/polycast/Spartech-Polycast-Solacryl-Monkey-Shine.pdf

Vitamin D Wiki is a useful collection of vitamin D information:
http://vitamindwiki.com/VitaminDWiki

Capacitive filters:

STETZERiZER Filter: http://www.stetzerelectric.com/

Greenwave Filter: http://www.greenwavefilters.com/

Useful electromagnetic websites are:

American Academy of Environmental Medicine was founded in 1965, and is an international association of physicians and other professionals interested in the clinical aspects of humans and their environment: http://aaemonline.org/

AntennaSearch Report: http://www.antennasearch.com/

Bioinitiative Report is a rationale for biologically-based public exposure standards for electromagnetic fields (ELF and RF): http://www.bioinitiative.org/

British Society for Ecological Medicine has existed as a professional body since 1983 and has made a major contribution to the integration of ecological principles into mainstream medicine in the UK: http://www.bsem.org.uk/

Canadians for Safe Technology: http://www.c4st.org/

Cellular Phone Task Force is dedicated to halting the expansion of wireless technology because it cannot be made safe: http://www.cellphonetaskforce.org/

Dr. Magda Havas, PhD, co-author of "Public Health SOS: The Shadow Side of the Wireless Revolution":

http://www.magdahavas.com/

Dr. Nina Pierpont is developing the health effects of wind turbines and infrasound: http://www.windturbinesyndrome.com/

Dr. Samuel Milham, author of "Dirty Electricity":

http://www.sammilham.com/

ElectroSensitivity UK is a website that aims to provide unbiased and balanced information to help those who have become sensitive to mobile and cordless phones, their masts, WiFi, and a multitude of common everyday electrical appliances: http://www.es-uk.info/

EMFacts Consultancy, founded in 1994 by Don Maisch, has produced a wide range of reports and papers dealing with various health issues related to human exposure to electromagnetic radiation: http://www.emfacts.com/

Environmental Health Center-Dallas, Texas, medically tests and treats human health problems including sensitivities to pollens, molds, dust, foods, chemicals, air (indoor/outdoor), water, electromagnetic sensitivity (EMF), and many more health problems as they relate to our environment: http://www.ehcd.com/

Environmental Radiation LLC offers the services to identify the modern invisible toxins that we are routinely exposed to and the know-how to rectify the problems.

http://www.environmentalradiation.com/

Guidelines of the Austrian Medical Association for the diagnosis and treatment of EMF related health problems and illnesses (EMF syndrome): http://freiburger-appell-2012.info/media/EMF%20Guideline%20OAK-AG%20%202012%2003%2003.pdf

Less EMF are a leading supplier in the USA of electromagnetic radiation products: http://www.lessemf.com/

Lloyd Burrell, Author of "Beating Electrical Sensitivity – The Path to Tread" and "Long Term EMF Protection – Start Feeling Better Today", has an excellent website on electromagnetic radiation exposures: http://www.electricsense.com/

Mast-Victims.org - An international community website for people suffering adverse health effects from mobile phone masts in the vicinity of their homes: http://www.mast-victims.org/

Medical Perspective on Environmental Sensitivities - Canadian Human Rights Commission: http://www.chrc-ccdp.gc.ca/sites/default/files/envsensitivity_en.pdf

OSCILLATORIUM: A gallery of images and maps, visual learning tools for the study of unnatural oscillations, non-ionizing electromagnetic fields, and their effects on living tissues and biodiverse systems: http://www.oscillatorium.com/

Powerwatch UK: http://www.powerwatch.org.uk/

Safe in School is documenting Electromagnetic Hypersensitivity in children: http://www.safeinschool.org/

Smart Meter Opposition Groups in the United States of America: http://www.takebackyourpower.net/directory/us/

Spaceweather: Current space weather conditions are available at: http://www.spaceweather.com/

WEEP - The Canadian initiative to stop wireless, electric, and electromagnetic pollution: http://www.weepinitiative.org/

World Health Organization (WHO) International Workshop on Electromagnetic Field Hypersensitivity: http://www.who.int/peh-emf/publications/reports/EHS_Proceedings_June2006.pdf

"The Internet is becoming the town square for the global village of tomorrow."

Bill Gates

EHS Groups

Facebook groups for health effects of electromagnetic radiation exposures:

- https://www.facebook.com/groups/661015143934586/ (B.C. WIRELESS-FREE ZONES)
- https://www.facebook.com/groups/citizensforsafetechnol ogy/
- https://www.facebook.com/groups/electromagneticsensit ivity/
- https://www.facebook.com/groups/486235528102748/ (Electro Sensitive Syndrome (ESS))
- https://www.facebook.com/groups/169495243194739/ (Electro-sensitivity Forum...)
- https://www.facebook.com/groups/EMFHarm/
- https://www.facebook.com/groups/emfSensitivity/
- https://www.facebook.com/groups/FriendOofDirtyElectr icityandEMFConquerors/
- https://www.facebook.com/groups/307214196137645/ (SMART Resistance UK)
- https://www.facebook.com/groups/675328022574090/ (UK Electrosensitives)
- https://www.facebook.com/groups/214991361950922/ (Victims of Wireless Technology Registry)
- https://www.facebook.com/groups/168893473164462/ (WEEP Initiative ~EHS Support)
- https://www.facebook.com/groups/571481532909496/ (WIRELESS FREE LIVING COMMUNITIES)

Yahoo Group:

- https://groups.yahoo.com/neo/groups/emfrefugee/info
  (EMF Refugee)

"Sensitivity to electromagnetic radiation is the emerging health problem of the 21st century. It is imperative health practitioners, governments, schools and parents learn more about it. The human health stakes are significant".

William Rea, MD

Twitter

Interesting Twitter news regarding biologically harmful environmental radiation exposures can be found here:

- https://twitter.com/4SafePhones
- https://twitter.com/4safeschools
- https://twitter.com/BanTXSmartMeter
- https://twitter.com/berkeleyprc
- https://twitter.com/blogBRHP
- https://twitter.com/BurbankACTION
- https://twitter.com/_C4ST
- https://twitter.com/CABTA
- https://twitter.com/CamillaRees
- https://twitter.com/CellPhonePain
- https://twitter.com/ChronicExposure
- https://twitter.com/Cleanwires
- https://twitter.com/cst_org
- https://twitter.com/davehubert
- https://twitter.com/DevraLeeDavis
- https://twitter.com/DianneKnight
- https://twitter.com/EHSsufferer
- https://twitter.com/ElectroSmog
- https://twitter.com/electrosmogs
- https://twitter.com/elliemarks
- https://twitter.com/emfanalysis

- https://twitter.com/EMFRadResearch
- https://twitter.com/EMFSafetyNet
- https://twitter.com/EMFStavanger
- https://twitter.com/emfwise
- https://twitter.com/EMRHABC
- https://twitter.com/emrpolicy
- https://twitter.com/EMRStop
- https://twitter.com/EMShield
- https://twitter.com/EnergyCanaries
- https://twitter.com/EnvironmentEMR
- https://twitter.com/eonnewsnet
- https://twitter.com/EVILSmartMeters
- https://twitter.com/FreqSensitive
- https://twitter.com/HandsFreeInfo
- https://twitter.com/info_KSTI
- https://twitter.com/janhaviii
- https://twitter.com/joshuanoahhart
- https://twitter.com/KillerRadiation
- https://twitter.com/KimPigSquash
- https://twitter.com/Lisanagy
- https://twitter.com/lloydburrell
- https://twitter.com/Microwave_Tower
- https://twitter.com/mobilewise
- https://twitter.com/newsomega
- https://twitter.com/No2SmartMeters
- https://twitter.com/NoBCsmartmeters
- https://twitter.com/NoBriarlakeTowr

- https://twitter.com/No_Radiation_4U
- https://twitter.com/NoRFIDinschools
- https://twitter.com/NoSmartMetersBC
- https://twitter.com/nosmartmeterlbk
- https://twitter.com/NOSMARTMETERSTX
- https://twitter.com/Notosmartmeters
- https://twitter.com/RFIDFreeSchools
- https://twitter.com/richardcriddle
- https://twitter.com/practicesafetek
- https://twitter.com/SafeinSchoolOrg
- https://twitter.com/SaferEMF
- https://twitter.com/saferphones
- https://twitter.com/SmartMeterAware
- https://twitter.com/smartmetermatrx
- https://twitter.com/Smartmeterno
- https://twitter.com/SmartMetersKill
- https://twitter.com/SmartMetersSuck
- https://twitter.com/SpyMeters
- https://twitter.com/stopbelltower
- https://twitter.com/StopSmartMeter
- https://twitter.com/stopsmeters
- https://twitter.com/stopsmetersaust
- https://twitter.com/StopSmrtMeterBC
- https://twitter.com/SustainableM
- https://twitter.com/TBYPfilm
- https://twitter.com/UK_EHS
- https://twitter.com/UnaStClair

- https://twitter.com/UnionRoots2Know
- https://twitter.com/vegosapien
- https://twitter.com/wannabewired
- https://twitter.com/wilcom_neha
- https://twitter.com/WiredChild
- https://twitter.com/WirelessFreeZn
- https://twitter.com/WirelessSmog
- https://twitter.com/WhoaTower
- https://twitter.com/whynotwired
- https://twitter.com/youcantsmartme

"Most people have no idea that OSHA is a ghost and has been so for years"

Devra Davis

Recommended Books and Films

The following books are recommended:

- An Electronic Silent Spring: Facing the Dangers and Creating Safe Limits by Katie Singer.

- Beating Electrical Sensitivity by Lloyd Burrell.

- Challenging the Chip: Labor Rights and Environmental Justice in the Global Electronics Industry by Ted Smith et al.

- Cross Currents by Dr. Robert O. Becker.

- Dirty Electricity by Samuel Milham.

- Disconnect: The Truth About Cell Phone Radiation, What the Industry Is Doing to Hide It, and How to Protect Your Family by Devra Davis.

- Doubt is Their Product: How Industry's Assault on Science Threatens Your Health by David Michaels.

- Electrical Forensics by Steven Magee.

- Electrocution of America: Is Your Utility Company Out to Kill You? by Russ Allen.

- Electromagnetic Fields by B. Blake Levitt.

- Electromagnetic Radiation Survival Guide - Step by Step Solutions - Protect Yourself & Family NOW! by Jonathan Halpern.

- Electromagnetic Sensitivity and Electromagnetic Hypersensitivity: A Summary by Michael Bevington.

- Healing is Voltage: The Handbook, 3rd Edition by Jerry L. Tennant.

- Health Forensics by Steven Magee.

- Light Forensics by Steven Magee.

- Light, Radiation, and You: How to Stay Healthy by John N. Ott.

- MOTORCYCLE CANCER? ELF EMF radiation truth exposed for rider safety by Randall Dale Chipkar.

- Public Health SOS: The Shadow Side Of The Wireless Revolution by Camilla Rees & Magda Havas.

- The Force by Lyn McLean.

- The Invisible Disease by Gunni Nordstrom.

- The Secret Life of Plants by Peter Thomkins & Christopher Bird.

- The Secret History of the War on Cancer by Devra Davis.

- Tracing EMFs in Building Wiring and Grounding by Karl Riley.

- Zapped by Ann Louise Gittleman.

The following documentaries are recommended viewing:

- Electrosensitive: Outliers in a Wireless World by Thomas Ball.

- Exploring the Spectrum by Dr. John Nash Ott.

- Full Signal: The Hidden Cost of Cell Phones by Talal Jabari.

- Microwaves, Science and Lies by Jean Hèches.

- Mobilize by Kevin Kunze.

- Resonance - Beings of Frequency by James Russell.

- Take Back Your Power by Josh del Sol.

- Windfall by Laura Israel.

"Radio frequency radiation and other forms of electromagnetic pollution are harmful at orders of magnitude well below existing guidelines. Science is one of the tools society uses to decide health policy. In the case of telecommunications equipment, such as cell phones, wireless networks, cell phone antennas, PDAs, and portable phones, the science is being ignored. Current guidelines urgently need to be re-examined by government and reduced to reflect the state of the science. There is an emerging public health crisis at hand and time is of the essence."

Magda Havas, PhD

CDC Cell Phone FAQ

Frequently Asked Questions about Cell Phones and Your Health: Most of us depend on cell phones every day. Some people wonder if cell phones can cause health problems. Here's what you should know about cell phones and your health.

Can using a cell phone cause cancer?

There is no scientific evidence that provides a definite answer to that question. Along with many organizations worldwide, **we recommend caution in cell phone use.** More research is needed before we know for sure if using cell phones causes cancer.

Do cell phones give off (emit) radiation?

Yes – cell phones and cordless phones use radio frequency radiation (RF) to send signals. RF is different from other types of radiation (like x-rays) that we know can be harmful. We don't know for sure if RF radiation from cell phones can cause health problems years later. **The International Agency for Research on Cancer (IARC) has classified RF radiation as a "possible human carcinogen." (A carcinogen is an agent that causes cancer.)**

Should people stop using cell phones?

Scientific studies are ongoing. **Someday cellphones may be found to cause health problems we are not aware of at this time.** However it is also important to consider the benefits of cell phones. They can be valuable in an urgent or emergency situation– and even save lives. If you are worried about cell phone use, follow the tips below.

Cell phone tips; To reduce radio frequency radiation near your body:

- Get a hands-free headset that connects directly to your phone.

- Use speaker-phone more often.

- If you have a pacemaker, keep cell phones at least 8 inches away from it.

Do cell phones cause health problems in children?

It's too soon to know for sure. Children who use cell phones – and continue to use them as they get older – are likely to be around RF for many years. **If RF does cause health problems, kids who use cell phones may have a higher chance of developing these problems in the future.**

What research is being done to learn more about cell phones and health?

Scientists are continuing to study the possible health effects of cell phone use. For example, the World Health Organization (WHO) is currently looking into how cell phones may affect:

- Some types of tumors (a lump or growth).

- Our eyes.

- Sleep.

- Memory.

- Headaches.

In the News: **Acoustic Neuroma. Scientists are looking into a possible link between cell phone use and certain types of tumor. One type is called an acoustic neuroma ("ah-COOS-tik nur-OH-ma"). This type of tumor grows on the nerve that connects the ear to the brain. It doesn't cause cancer, but it**

may lead to other health problems, like hearing loss. Another type scientists are looking into is called a glioma ("glee-OH-ma"). This is a tumor found in the brain or central nervous system of the body.

Where can I get more information about cell phones and health?

For more information, visit:

The Federal Communications Commission

World Health Organization

The Food and Drug Administration

Contact Us:

Centers for Disease Control and Prevention, 1600 Clifton Rd, Atlanta, GA 30333

800-CDC-INFO(800-232-4636)

Page last reviewed: June 9, 2014

Page last updated: June 9, 2014

"The U.S. spends over $2 trillion dollars on health care each year, of which about 78% is from people with chronic illnesses, without adequately exploring and understanding what factors —including EMF/RF—contribute to imbalances in peoples' bodies' in the first place. After reading The BioInitiative Report, it should come as no surprise to policymakers, given the continually increasing levels of EMF/RF exposures in our environment, that close to 50% of Americans now live with a chronic illness. I grieve for people who needlessly suffer these illnesses and hold out the hope that our government leaders will become more cognizant of the role electromagnetic factors are playing in disease, health care costs and the erosion of quality of life and productivity in America."

Camilla Rees, MBA

Signs & Symptoms of RWS & EHS

Radio frequency power level exposures exceeding the FCC guidelines for tissue heating:

- Skin feeling warm.
- Skin burning.
- Organ damage.
- Eye damage.
- Flu-like symptoms.

Short term exposure to biologically harmful radio waves leads to:

- Extensive fatigue that leads to apathy.

Long term exposure to biologically harmful radio waves leads to:

- Neurasthenia symptoms.

Prolonged exposure to biologically harmful radio waves leads to:

- Dull pressure in the head.
- Headaches that become intolerable.
- Depression.
- Inferiority.
- Complaining.
- Arguing.
- Uncertainty in dealing with others.

Exposure to cell phone towers, cell phones, Wi-Fi, domestic wireless devices and radio frequency transmitting utility meters is known to cause:

- Fatigue.

- Sleep disturbance.

- Headaches.

- Feeling of discomfort.

- Difficulty in concentrating.

- Depression.

- Memory loss.

- Visual disruptions.

- Irritability.

- Hearing disruptions.

- Skin problems.

- Cardiovascular.

- Dizziness.

- Loss of appetite.

- Movement difficulties

- Nausea.

Dr. Erwin Schliephake found that the symptoms of Radio Wave Sickness would resolve shortly after removal of the radio transmitter. In general, he found that low powered radio frequency (RF) would cause tranquilizing effects and high powered RF created irritation. The sensitivity was person dependent.

Cold sores are the radiation alarm system of the human body. If you are having frequent cold sores then you should check out your environment for the various forms of radiation exposures. You may ultimately need to move home, change your job or switch to a new occupation to clear them up.

Hot skin with general aches and pains are the symptoms of a solar radiation overload condition. This is not sunburn, but a sustained daily over-exposure to high intensity light. It is easily cured by reducing your daily exposure to daylight.

Sensitivity to blue light appears to be a blue light deficiency condition that is remedied by looking out to the polar sky at the horizon. Approximately half an hour of "Horizon Polar Sky Fatigue Therapy" appears to clear up the blue light deficiency condition.

"We're in a dangerous world"

Professor Martin Pall

Recommended Test Meters

Most people are finding that they are being affected by radio waves or magnetic fields. The entry level meters for these two fields are regarded as:

- Battery Powered Portable AM Radio – Detects fields when tuned into static (no radio station).

- Cornet ED78S – Magnetic and radio frequency meter.

For many people, they add the following meters:

- Trifield 100XE – Magnetic, electric and microwave field meter.

- Telephone Recording Pickup Coil & Amplified Speaker – Detects stray currents and magnetic fields.

- Stetzerizer Microsurge Meter – For detecting dirty electricity.

For stray voltage work, people use the following personal computer data logging meters:

- TekPower TP4000ZC – For measuring temperature.

- UNI-T UT61D – For measuring true RMS maximum and minimum values of stray voltage.

- UNI-T UT61E – For measuring positive and negative peak values of stray voltage.

Professionals may use some of the following meters in addition to the above:

- Three Axis Radio Frequency Meter 10 MHz to 8 GHz (Tenmars TM-196, TES 593 or Extech 480846) – Reads ambient radio frequency radiation power levels. Not accurate on millisecond pulsed radio frequency radiation sources.

- Gigahertz Solutions HFEW35C – Specialized meter for measuring pulsed radio frequency radiation, such as from radio frequency transmitting utility meters and RADAR.

- RF Explorer Model 3G Combo — Handheld / USB RF Spectrum Analyzer.

- Whistler XTR-445 Battery Operated LASER/RADAR Detector.

- Gigahertz Solutions NFA1000 – Magnetic field meter.

- Gigahertz Solutions Magnetostatic Probe MS-NFA – For measuring constant magnetic fields that you find around solar photovoltaic modules and wiring.

- Gigahertz Solutions Electrostatic Probe ES-NFA – For measuring electrostatic charges on surfaces, such as carpets.

- Owon SDS6062V Battery Powered Digital Oscilloscope with Fast Fourier Transform (FFT) Function.

"Benjamin Franklin may have discovered electricity, but it was the man who invented the meter who made the money."

Earl Wilson

Acknowledgments

This book was influenced by:

- Claudia Sandoval M.S.W. for her wisdom on trees and how it relates in the social environment.

- Elizabeth Kelley MA for sharing her two decades of extensive experience working as a public heath advocate on the potential health risks of electromagnetic radiation.

- My neighbors for their understanding and assistance with my biological experiments.

- Dr. John Nash Ott for his extensive research into health, light, and radiation. His lasting legacy of publications was a wonderful gift to the next generation:

  o My Ivory Cellar; [the story of time-lapse photography].

  o Health and Light: The Extraordinary Study That Shows How Light Affects Your Health and Emotional Well Being.

  o Light, Radiation, and You: How to Stay Healthy.

  o Color and Light: Their Effects on Plants, Animals and People.

  o Exploring the Spectrum: The Effects of Natural and Artificial Light on Living Organisms.

- The numerous groups that have formed around the world to discuss and research the condition of Electromagnetic Hypersensitivity.

- The many people who have posted comments on the StevenMageeBooks research channel on YouTube. These have really helped progress research into electromagnetic radiation.

- The numerous people and companies who are referenced in this book that have worked diligently to bring the important science of environmental health to the masses.

"Help others achieve their dreams and you will achieve yours."

Les Brown

About the Author

Steven started his career at one of the largest university research and teaching hospitals in Europe. Working in the electrical engineering group, he obtained a Bachelors Degree with Honors in Electrical and Electronic Engineering. Human health was a strong draw and he moved into the biomedical team, serving the regions hospitals. During this time he developed a fascination for human illness and disease and the causes of it, many of which were not understood.

He joined the Isaac Newton Group of Telescopes in 1999 and went to live in La Palma. La Palma is part of the Canary Islands, governed by Spain. During this time he worked with the leading European astronomers and developed his astronomical and optics skills. He became fluent in Spanish and their culture.

In 2001 he became a Chartered Electrical Engineer and joined the W. M. Keck Observatory in Hawaii. This was the world's leading astronomical facility and home to the world's two largest segmented mirror telescopes. Steven developed segmented optics and interferometry skills while working alongside world leading astronomers. During this time Steven constructed his own off-grid solar powered home in the last of the traditional Hawaiian fishing villages in Miloli'i, Hawaii. He learned Hawaiian Pidgin English and the Hawaiian culture during his time there.

In 2006, Steven became the Director of the MDM Observatory in Sells, Arizona, USA. Working for Columbia University and later, Dartmouth College, he developed the facility to modern standards. He learned an appreciation of the native Americans and their culture from the Tohono O'odham Nation.

In 2008, Steven joined the solar power revolution that was sweeping the USA and commissioned the largest CIGS thin film solar photovoltaic installation in the world.

A year later he commissioned the largest solar photovoltaic power plant in the USA. The system rated power was quoted as 25,000,000 watts AC with over 90,500 solar modules that were mounted to 158 single-axis tracker systems in three hundred acres of land.

He went on to develop the solar photovoltaic team for a large international company.

In 2010 he started to research radiation and publish the leading books on the subject.

"All truths are easy to understand once they are discovered; the point is to discover them."

Galileo Galilei

Author Contact

I hope that you found the book informative and please let me know if you have any questions or comments. I can be contacted through the StevenMageeBooks channel on www.youtube.com.

I am a consultant in the areas that I research at Environmental Radiation LLC and please feel free to contact me for any help or assistance. This is the website:

http://www.environmentalradiation.com/

You can follow the @EnvironmentEMR Twitter feed at:

https://twitter.com/EnvironmentEMR

The Facebook page is:

https://www.facebook.com/EnvironmentEMR

You may find my other books useful:

Solar Photovoltaic

- **Complete Solar Photovoltaics for Residential, Commercial, and Utility Systems:** Steven Magee has combined his three top selling books on solar power systems into one edition. Complete Solar Photovoltaics will train you on solar photovoltaics and show you how to design grid connected solar photovoltaic power systems. Operations and maintenance is detailed to enable you to have a complete understanding of solar photovoltaics from start to finish.

- **Solar Photovoltaics for Consumers, Utilities, and Investors:** This book details solar photovoltaic systems for consumers, utilities and investors. This would encompass residential, commercial and utility systems that are connected to the utility grid. There is a discussion of the different technologies available for the consumer and their advantages and disadvantages. For the utilities, there is invaluable advice on planning and constructing large projects. For the investor, forward looking statements try to predict the future of solar photovoltaics.

- **Solar Photovoltaic Training for Residential, Commercial, and Utility Systems:** This book details solar photovoltaic training for those who are interested in this area and also for those who are already working in the field. This would encompass residential, commercial, and utility systems that are connected to the utility grid. It is a comprehensive overview of a rapidly growing world of solar photovoltaic power generation technology.

- **Solar Photovoltaic Design for Residential, Commercial, and Utility Systems:** This book details how to design reliable solar photovoltaic power generation systems from a residential system, progressing to a commercial system, and finishing at the largest utility power generation systems. By following the guidelines in this book and your local solar photovoltaic electrical codes, you will be able to design trouble free solar power systems that give many years of reliable operation. When designed well, solar photovoltaic power generation is an excellent source of electrical power that results in much lower electricity bills, the power company will even refund you for the excess energy generated by your system if it is large enough. Building a grid tied solar power system is a relatively easy task. Given the large amount of government and electrical utility financial incentives that are available, it is a great time to join in the solar power revolution that is taking place in the world today.

- **Solar Photovoltaic Operation and Maintenance for Residential, Commercial, and Utility Systems:** This book details how to operate and maintain residential, commercial, and utility solar photovoltaic systems that are connected to the utility grid. By following the guidelines in this book you will be able to operate and maintain solar power systems that should give many years of reliable operation. Invaluable trouble shooting advice will aid in returning your system to full operation in the event of a problem.

- **Solar Photovoltaic DC Calculations for Residential, Commercial, and Utility Systems:** This book details how to run calculations for the DC circuit of solar photovoltaic systems. This would encompass residential, commercial, and utility systems that are connected to the utility grid. It covers the range of conditions that solar photovoltaic modules are exposed to throughout the year and shows how to incorporate these into an effective DC circuit that is well designed and reliable.

- **Solar Photovoltaic Resource for Residential, Commercial, and Utility Systems:** This book is a resource of information that is used in the solar photovoltaic field. This would encompass residential, commercial, and utility systems that are connected to the utility grid. It is a comprehensive collection of notes, diagrams, pictures and charts for a rapidly growing world of solar photovoltaic power generation technology. This book is illustrated in color.

Solar

- **Solar Irradiance and Insolation for Power Systems:** This book is a resource of information that is used in the solar power generation field. This would encompass residential, commercial, and utility systems that are connected to the utility grid. It is a comprehensive collection of notes, diagrams, pictures, and charts for a rapidly growing world of solar photovoltaic power generation technology. This book is illustrated in color.

- **Solar Site Selection for Power Systems:** This book is a comprehensive collection of images, diagrams, and notes that document the effects of light and heat in the solar power generation field. This would encompass residential, commercial, and utility systems that are connected to the utility grid. This is essential information for a rapidly growing world of solar power generation technology. This book is illustrated in color.

Architecture

- **Solar Reflections for Architects, Engineers, and Human Health:** This book is a comprehensive collection of images, diagrams, and notes that document the effects of sunlight in architecture. This is essential information for architects, engineers, and the medical profession. The discovery of the "Multiple-Sun" effect in architecture is detailed and this book is illustrated in color.

Human Health

- **Curing Electromagnetic Hypersensitivity:** Steven Magee received a biologically toxic electromagnetic radiation exposure in 2009. This led to the realization that he had been displaying the symptoms of low level radiation sickness for many years. This book documents his journey into the radiation sickness condition of Electromagnetic Hypersensitivity and the many steps that he took to cure it.

- **Solar Radiation – A Cause of Illness and Cancer?** Illness and cancers have become part of our modern culture. It has been discovered that extremely high levels of man-made solar radiation exist in modern society. Could this be the one of the causes of illness and cancers? This book examines the increase in solar radiation and applies it to human health.

- **Solar Radiation, Global Warming, and Human Disease:** This book examines the modern development of the Earth and the potential impacts on global warming and human disease. The destruction of the forests for modern agricultural use appears to have effects that are not fully understood and these are explored. Radiation deficiency and radiation overloading are investigated to see if they are factors in many illnesses and diseases.

- **Toxic Light:** Toxic Light takes a look at the light pollution that may be in your local environment and relates it to the health problems that it may cause. Light in the human environment is only just starting to be understood and something as innocent as your sunglasses may be able to make you ill! There are many examples of commonplace items in your environment that may have the ability to affect your health. Get ready for enlightenment about the most important human nutrient of light!

- **Toxic Health:** Toxic Health takes a look at the pollution that may be in your local environment and relates it to the health problems that it can cause. Pollution in the human environment is only just starting to be understood and something as innocent as light may be able to make you really ill! There are many examples of commonplace items in your environment that may have the ability to affect your health. In particular, we will investigate if modern city life is the most toxic thing of all to the modern human!

- **Toxic Electricity:** Random aches and pains? Fatigue? Insomnia? Facial pains? Irregular heartbeats? Sick kids? Relationship problems? Blotchy skin? Anxiety? Toxic electricity takes a look at the electrical system and asks the question: Is this one of the most toxic endeavors that humanity has ever engaged in?

Forensics

- **Electrical Forensics:** Electrical Forensics examines the many aspects of electricity, electronics and wireless communications that may lead to unusual behaviors to occur in humans. Electromagnetic interference is well known for its ability to affect mental functioning and human health. Electrical Forensics demonstrates how to identify toxic electromagnetic environments that may be the root cause of accidents and crimes.

- **Health Forensics:** Health Forensics examines the many aspects of modern society that may lead to unusual behaviors to occur in humans. Modern society has adopted habits that are well known for their ability to affect mental functioning and human health. Health Forensics demonstrates how to identify toxic human environments that may be the root cause of accidents and crimes.

- **Light Forensics:** Light Forensics examines the many aspects of modern lighting that may lead to unusual behaviors to occur in humans. Modern society has adopted optical products that are well known for their ability to affect mental functioning and human health. Light Forensics demonstrates how to identify toxic light that may be the root cause of accidents and crimes.

Religion

- **Solar Radiation, the Book of Revelations, and the Era of Light – Part 1:** Welcome to the Era of Light! Light has long been known to be essential nourishment for the human body. We will explore the different types of light that are present on Earth and relate it to human health and nature. Light is discussed extensively in the Bible and we will see if we can associate our findings to it.

Finally, we will investigate if the Industrial Revolution has created the ultimate toxin of poisonous sunlight!

Professional

- **Engineering Science and Education Journal Volume: 11, Issue: 4, Active Control Systems for Large Segmented Optical Mirrors:** A new generation of optical telescopes is on the drawing board. These will be true giants with primary mirrors having a diameter of up to 100 meters. The technology that will enable this revolution to take place was developed at the W. M. Keck Observatory in Hawaii, where the world's largest segmented mirrors are in daily use. This article looks at how the W. M. Keck Observatory proved the mirror technology that will be behind this new generation of telescopes.

Electromagnetic Frequency Research

- **7.83Hz Schumann Resonance to the Eighth Harmonic:** This is the research soundtrack that was developed for the books Toxic Health and Health Forensics. It contains harmonics of the original 7.83 Hertz fundamental frequency through to the eighth harmonic. It is designed to be used with electrical headphones as you are applying an electromagnetic wave to the human brain. Tracks with harmonics 1, 2 or 3 may not be audible, but do produce the electromagnetic wave from the coils inside the headphones. The soundtrack is aimed at people who want to research the health effects of electrical headphones and Schumann Resonance electromagnetic waves.

You can search "Steven Magee Books" for the very latest publications.

www.youtube.com videos supporting the ideas in the books can be found by searching: StevenMageeBooks

"Life-transforming ideas have always come to me through books."

Bell Hooks

Book Reviews

Health Forensics rated 5 out of 5 stars.

Review by Ann on April 29, 2014 titled "A Must Read for Your Health!"

If you care about staying healthy or suffer with chronic illness, I recommend reading Health Forensics and other books written by Steven Magee. He has not only researched extensively on the subject of Electromagnetic Hypersensitivity (EHS) but has experienced the ill effects of it himself. So he knows firsthand. I found Health Forensics to be written in a way that would be easy for anyone to read. The author gave very clear steps on how we can protect ourselves from the modern day hazards in our environment. Some of them are right in plain view and we don't even realize it. In the book, he has shared invaluable information that, I believe, can help those of us who are already suffering from EHS, prevent others from being adversely affected, and give us a way to live healthier lives. Also, I would recommend this book for those who may have lyme disease, autoimmune disease, immune deficiency, lupus, fibromyalgia, chronic fatigue, just to name a few, or any unexplainable and persistent symptoms. Thank you Steven Magee for your willingness to help others.

Electrical Forensics rated 5 out of 5 stars.

Review by John Puccetti on October 27, 2013 titled "Dangers of electricity"

Steven has made many of the health problems of our century known in his book. But what will we do with this information? We live in a corporate dictatorship that masquerades as democracy.

Toxic Electricity rated 5 out of 5 stars.

Review by Sam Wieder on December 13, 2013 titled "A Most Illuminating, Educational, and Helpful Book"

Toxic Electricity provides a clear and comprehensive description of the many ways in which electrical fields impact human health and offers simple steps that anyone can take to live a more vibrant life in our electrically toxic world. The author does a masterful job of presenting some fairly complex concepts in a way that is easily understandable. Reading this book will give you a deeper understanding of how unseen radiation in your living and working environment may be impacting you. If you've been battling different health challenges or are chronically tired for no apparent reason, this book may very well open your eyes to some answers that will help you regain your health and your life.

Toxic Light rated 4 out of 5 Stars.

Review by John Puccetti on January 2, 2014 titled "Very technical".

I recommend you read "Tesla a man out of time" before you read this book. It is hard to grasp how much is wrong with radio frequencies and the electric grid and smart meters unless you really do some research first. But it is a wake up call to us all. Well worth reading.

Curing Electromagnetic Hypersensitivity rated 5 out of 5 Stars.

Review by Mr. Steven Phillips on November 20, 2014 titled "Five Stars".

Excellent book! Thank you...

"A good, sympathetic review is always a wonderful surprise."

Joyce Carol Oates

Made in the USA
San Bernardino, CA
20 January 2015